Learning Theory and Stuttering Therapy

Learning Theory and

Stuttering Therapy

Edited by Hugo H. Gregory

Northwestern University Press

Evanston   1968

The publication of this book has been aided by
a grant from the Speech Foundation of America

Hugo H. Gregory is Associate Professor of Speech
Pathology and Director of Stuttering Programs,
Northwestern University

Preface

THERE HAS BEEN A STEADILY DEVELOPING INTEREST in the interpretation of stuttering behavior using a psychological learning theory frame of reference, with particular emphasis on the contributions of Hull, Miller, Mowrer, and Skinner. Thus, it has become increasingly essential for the speech pathologist working with stutterers to have a rather extensive comprehension of learning theory.

This book grew out of lectures presented at a symposium, "Principles of Learning and the Management of Stuttering," held at Northwestern University in the summer of 1965. The participants revised their own chapters, and the concluding chapter was written during the first six months of 1967.

Interest in this topic has been intensified by the recent emphasis within psychology on behavior therapy—the application of learning theory to the treatment of psychological disorders. Behavior therapists and speech pathologists have found in the problem of stuttering a disorder which—due to the nature of its development, observability, and susceptibility to modification—is of mutual interest. The purposes of this series of lectures were to focus attention upon basic principles of learning which have been related to the onset and development of stuttering and to appraise the application of these learning theory concepts, alone or in conjunction with other approaches, to the treatment of stuttering.

The literature on the psychology of learning is immense. Even the literature reporting stuttering research (e.g., that on consistency, adaptation, and spontaneous recovery) and therapeutic procedures related to psychological principles of learning is relatively extensive. Therefore, it is the objective of this book, as it was in the symposium, to cite and discuss the essentials of these developments with especial reference to the implications for stuttering therapy. The reader whose interest is aroused by these papers will want to acquaint himself with the work of other clinicians and researchers who are mentioned therein, and whose publications are cited in the bibliography at the end of the text. I have made a particular effort in the concluding chapter to direct the reader to still other significant references.

Mowrer's first chapter, which is historical in organization and which attempts to synthesize the traditional and contemporary theories of learning in terms of the revised two-factor theory, was selected as the point of departure, since it encompasses most of the theoretical work related to stuttering. I discuss the differences in approach and emphasis between Dollard and Miller, Skinner (whose contributions have also influenced speech pathology), and Mowrer in the concluding chapter.

In the second chapter, Murray describes social learning and personality in terms of behavior change, with special reference to the Dollard and Miller analysis of learning. He shows how learning theory has been utilized in traditional and newer forms of psychotherapy. His discussion establishes a foundation for the chapters by Luper, Mowrer, Sheehan, Williams, and myself, that consider learning concepts with reference to the specific types of behavior change desired in stuttering therapy. In the last chapter, I have summarized some of the main points made in the book, delineated areas of agreement and disagreement, indicated possible conclusions and implications, and pointed to significant contributions which were not covered specifically in the symposium.

Many people made this book possible. Harold Westlake, former Chairman of the Department of Communicative Disorders, and James H. McBurney, Dean of the School of Speech at Northwestern, supported the plan for a symposium on this subject. David Rutherford, the present Chairman of the Department of Communicative Disorders, has provided helpful advice during the period of preparing the material for publication. David Dickson made the arrangements with the Vocational Rehabilitation Administration to provide scholarships for the symposium. Mrs. Elizabeth Ruddick was of great assistance in supervising the preparation of typescripts made from tape recordings of the symposium sessions.

I am indebted to my wife, Carolyn, for the editorial assistance and encouragement which she provided. Gratitude is also expressed to George Yacorzynski, Head of the Division of Psychology, Northwestern Medical School, who has encouraged my interest in the psychological aspects of speech disorders.

I want to acknowledge our appreciation to the Speech Foundation of America for the grant which covered the cost of typesetting this book. The Speech Foundation has contributed significantly to the prevention and treatment of stuttering by arranging opportunities for authorities in the field to meet together, discuss principles and procedures, and communicate with other practicing clinicians through the publication and distribution of six booklets during the last ten years. In making the grant in connection with this volume, Malcolm Fraser, Director of the Speech Foundation, said, "We hope this publication will help to spread information which will be of value in the treatment of this problem."

Last, but certainly not least, I want to express my appreciation to the authors who participated in the symposium and this subsequent publication. I am also grateful to them for their comments on the concluding chapter of the book.

Evanston, Illinois
August, 1967

H. H. G.

Contents

CONTENTS

List of Figures and Tables

Learning Theory and Stuttering Therapy

I

O. HOBART MOWRER

A Résumé of Basic Principles

of Learning

THE BEGINNING OF THE TWENTIETH CENTURY found American psychology undergoing a major transformation.[1] Since its founding as an independent science, some twenty-five years earlier, psychology had been largely preoccupied with "the study of consciousness, *per se,*" and its method was mainly that of introspection. Some systematic knowledge was thus acquired, especially as regards sensation and perception; but,

1. Editor's note: The material in this chapter, which is a summary of the developments presented in O. H. Mowrer, *Learning Theory and Behavior* (New York: John Wiley, 1960), was first published in Chap. I, "Resume and Introduction," of Mowrer's book, *Learning Theory and the Symbolic Processes* (New York: John Wiley, 1960). The reader who desires a more detailed consideration of this material and of Mowrer's contributions relating learning theory to the symbolic processes should consult both of these companion volumes.

Appreciation is expressed to John Wiley & Sons, Inc., for granting permission to reproduce selected sections of the chapter by Dr. Mowrer.

for the most part, the approach had proved limited and unproductive. This was particularly true of the psychology of learning.

Already, in 1896, Dewey had predicted that the New Psychology would be based upon the concept of the reflex arc—a prediction which proved to be well founded. Soon the work of Pavlov on "conditioned reflexes" was to arouse world-wide interest, and Thorndike was to introduce a theory of habit which, in a rather different sense, was equally reflexological.

The psychology of introspection (or so-called Structuralism) had been concerned with consciousness. Pavlov and Thorndike were concerned with objectively observable stimuli and responses. It was therefore not surprising that Watson (1914, 1919) should have coined and popularized the name, "Behaviorism," for the new movement.

THE FIRST TWO-FACTOR OR TWO-PROCESS CONCEPTION OF LEARNING

Although they were alike in that they were both behavioristic (and essentially "reflexological"), the views of Pavlov and those of Thorndike were in other respects quite different. Learning, as Pavlov conceived it, was entirely a matter of stimulus substitution. By the paired presentation or occurrence of two stimuli—an originally neutral, or "meaningless," one with another which already has the capacity to elicit a particular reaction—this reaction, according to Pavlov, gets connected with, or "conditioned" to, the formerly neutral stimulus. And since, in order for this process to take place, the originally neutral (ineffective) stimulus must occur first, somewhat in advance of the other (already effective) stimulus, the originally neutral stimulus may be said to act as a *signal;* so that, in conditioning, the organism learns to respond to signals, as well as to the things thus *signified*. Hence, it is understandable why Pavlov stressed the adaptive, life-preserving implications of this type of learning or behavior change.

In contrast, Thorndike saw learning as a matter of *response substitution*. It was not, he believed, so much a matter of an organism's coming to make the *same* response to a *new* stimulus as it was of its coming to make a *new* response to the *same* stimulus. If, for example, a particular stimulus (such as hunger) causes an animal to make a response which is rewarding (hunger-reducing), well and good: the connection, or "bond," between that stimulus and that response ought to be, and

4

presumably is, strengthened. But what a misfortune it would be if an organism kept repeating a useless or actively harmful response! Obviously organisms need and apparently have a device for getting rid of, or "disconnecting," such responses. This Thorndike called punishment or "stamping-out." Thus it is, reasoned Thorndike, that if one response to a particular stimulus does not work or works adversely, the organism can get rid of it, and, through "trial and error," find and fixate a better one.

Here, then, were two almost diametrically opposed conceptions of how learning operates, with a body of scientific as well as commonplace observations to support *each* of them. Psychologists, here in America and the world over, either "took sides" and sought to defend one position to the exclusion of the other or wondered, if, despite their seeming incompatibility, they might not both be true. The latter possibility is what may be termed the first *two-factor* or *two-process* conception of learning.

In 1932, E. C. Tolman published a book in which he took the position that all learning is *sign* learning, i.e., that it is simply a matter of new meanings or "cognitions," rather than overt responses, getting connected to appropriate stimuli. Given such a change in the "cognitive structure" or "psychological field" of the learner, more or less appropriate changes in behavior were assumed, somehow, to follow. Just how mere "knowledge" could instigate and control behavior was never fully explicated, a fact that prompted Guthrie (1952) to remark that Tolman's theory left the subject "lost in thought" instead of getting him to his goal.

Roughly a decade later, Clark L. Hull (1943), eschewing the subjectivism which Tolman (while still calling himself a Behaviorist) had allowed to creep into his theory, made an effort to unify the observations of Pavlov and Thorndike in a different way. Whereas Tolman had taken conditioning (he called it *sign* learning) as a basic and tried to derive trial-and-error behavior therefrom, Hull, turning the tables, took trial-and-error (Thorndikian) learning as basic and tried to make conditioning a by-product thereof.

Here it will not be necessary to indicate just how Hull approached this task or wherein his endeavor was unsuccessful. It will suffice to say that in 1947, the present writer, incorporating the research and thinking of a number of investigators, suggested a *second* version of two-factor theory (actually the first to carry this designation), which continued to posit a fundamental distinction between sign learning, on the one hand, and

5

solution learning on the other, but which also involved certain important departures from the way in which Pavlov and Thorndike had, respectively, defined them.

THE SECOND VERSION OF THE TWO-FACTOR PROCESS POSITION

When a buzzer sounds in the presence of a laboratory animal and the animal then receives a brief but moderately painful electric shock, we can be sure that the reaction of *fear,* originally aroused by the shock, will, after a few pairings of buzzer and shock, start occurring to the buzzer alone. Here the buzzer becomes a *sign* that shock is imminent, but no "solution" is yet in sight. Only when the subject, now motivated by the secondary (acquired, conditioned) drive of fear, starts behaving (as opposed to merely feeling) is he likely to hit upon some response which will "turn off" the danger signal and enable the subject to avert the shock. This, however, is no longer conditioning, or stimulus substitution, but habit formation. Here it seems that the subject first learns to *be afraid* and then what to *do* about the fear. These stages or steps were assumed to involve two separate and distinct *kinds* of learning: sign learning, i.e., the process whereby the fear gets shifted from the unconditioned to the conditioned stimulus; *and* solution learning, i.e., the process whereby an organism acquires the correct, effective instrumental response needed to lessen or eliminate the fear.[2]

This revised "two-factor" or "two-step" way of thinking about learning had some important advantages, chief among which is that it pro-

2. Editor's note: Wischner (1950) refers to this type of learning (known as instrumental avoidance training) in describing stuttering as a learned anxiety reaction system. He hypothesizes that noxious stimuli (disapproval by parents, teachers, etc., of a child's behavior) elicits anxiety (secondary drive) in the child, which brings about a disintegration of speech or "motivates the child to activity designed to avoid the noxious stimulation" (p. 329). Generalization occurs and sounds, words, and situations, as well as reactions of persons, become noxious stimulus cues for anxiety. Behavior such as the avoidance of words and situations is reinforced by anxiety reduction. Likewise, the stuttering speech behavior is reinforced as it is closely associated with anxiety reduction. Wischner points out, on the other hand, that obviously stuttering is also punishing to the speaker. To explain the relationship between the effects of reward and punishment in this case, he refers to Mowrer and Ullman's (1945) hypothesis as follows:

. . . if an act has two consequences . . . the one rewarding and the other punishing . . . which would be strictly equal if simultaneous, the influence of these consequences upon later performance of that act will vary depending upon the order in which they occur. If the punishing consequence comes first

vides an improved theory of "punishment." If an external, experimenter-controlled stimulus, like a buzzer, acquires the capacity to arouse fear as a result of having been paired with electric shock (or some other form of painful stimulation), would there not also be a form of fear conditioning which would occur when a shock follows something the subject *does?* Thorndike had assumed that when a stimulus-response sequence is followed by punishment, the latter acts in such a way as to *weaken* the pathway between stimulus and response, just as reward was supposed to strengthen this "connection." But it is obvious, even to casual observation, that the most immediate and reliable "effect" of behavior is neither punishment nor reward but, rather, the stimuli (sensations) associated with the occurrence of the behavior itself. Now if these response-correlated forms of stimulation are followed by an event such as electric shock, they will, by the principle of conditioning, themselves become capable of arousing fear, which can be allayed only if the subject *inhibits* the response which arouses them. In other words, if a response has been "punished," when the subject later starts to repeat that response, it will arouse proprioceptive, tactile, visual, or other forms of stimulation which will act as "danger signals" and will tend, through the fear they elicit, to block the response.

This interpretation of punishment was an improvement over Thorndike's stamping-out conception thereof, for it took into account the possibility of *conflict.* If a punishment acted as Thorndike supposed, then a habit, when subjected to punishment, would quietly fade away, deteriorate; whereas we know that living organisms do not give up established modes of gratification without a struggle. The notion that punishment causes fear to become connected to response-correlated stimuli is compatible with the observed facts and provides common ground, which had not existed before, between learning theory and clinical psychology.

Although "avoidance" learning was first studied in situations in which

---

and the reinforcing one later, the difference will be in favor of the inhibition. But if the rewarding consequence comes first and the punishing one later, the difference will be in favor of the reinforcement.

Wischner concluded:

It would seem, then, that in the case of stuttering behavior, though there may be both reward and punishment, the initial consequence is probably that of reinforcement due to tension reduction. According to the Mowrer-Ullman hypothesis, this would result in fixation of the non-integrative stuttering behavior (pp. 331–32).

the "warning" stimulus comes from the external environment, it was soon evident that, in principle, the situation is no different where the warning stimulus or stimuli are inherently associated with the subject's own activity. In the one case, fear gets conditioned to an independent stimulus or situation which the subject can perhaps flee from or manage in some other way, while in the other the fear gets conditioned to *response-aroused* stimuli which can occur only when a particular response occurs and can best be eliminated by cessation of the activity in question. Both of the forms of behavior cited involve "avoidance" but, in the one case, avoidance by "doing something" and, in the other, by not "doing something." In the one situation the subject may be said to get "punished" if he *does not* perform a particular response, whereas in the other he gets punished only if he *does* perform some specified response. The first may be termed *active* avoidance learning and the second, *passive* avoidance learning.

Here, clearly, is a way of thinking which has "power": by means of the same principles (fear conditioning followed by solution learning), one can account for two such seemingly diverse phenomena as flight and behavior inhibition. But there are also some inherent weaknesses; and in order to see these most clearly, it will be desirable to note the salient ways in which this second version of two-factor learning theory differed from the first. The first version had taken the views of both Pavlov and Thorndike more or less at face value, whereas the second version made certain important modifications. Pavlov had completely by-passed the problem of motivation and had tried to derive a wholly objective science of behavior from the concept of stimulus-substitution; in the second two-factor theory, it was assumed that what conditioning does, pre-eminently, is to attach *fears* to formerly neutral (independent or response-dependent) stimuli and that these fears then instigate trial-and-error behavior along lines very similar to those suggested by Thorndike. However, trial-and-error theory was also modified in two important ways: (1) whereas Thorndike had been interested almost exclusively in primary drives, such as hunger and thirst, the new two-factor position stressed the possibility of trial-and-error learning in response to secondary, as well as primary, drives; and (2), on the assumption that fears (once conditioned) may act as motivators and their reduction as reinforcers, a new conception of punishment (as well as active avoidance) emerged which was very different from the one advocated by Thorndike.

The two major weaknesses in the second version of two-factor learning theory were (a) that it did not adequately deal with what is now known as secondary reinforcement and (b) that it continued to accept, essentially unmodified, Thorndike's "bond" (reflexological) theory of habit.

REVISED TWO-FACTOR THEORY (THIRD VERSION)

Many years ago, Pavlov and his collaborators demonstrated what they called *second-order* salivary conditioning. If, for example, a blinking light is presented just before a hungry dog receives a bit of food, the salivary response which the food elicits (more or less reflexly) "moves forward" and starts to occur to the light alone. This is the familiar phenomenon of having one's "mouth water" at the sight, smell, or sound of food and represents what Pavlov called *first-order* conditioning. Then it was found, to continue with the same laboratory example, that the light, once the salivary response has been conditioned to it, can be paired with a *new* stimulus, e.g., the ticking of a metronome, and that, by this means, the salivary response can be transferred to the sound of the metronome, without the latter having ever been paired with the "primary" or original reinforcer, food. In other words, Pavlov showed that once the salivary response has been conditioned to a "first-order" conditioned stimulus, that stimulus can serve as the "unconditioned" stimulus for "second-order" conditioning.

Then, somewhat later, particularly as the result of researches in this country, it was found that a first-order conditioned stimulus can serve as a "secondary reinforcer" (the terminology is unfortunate but now conventional) in yet another sense. Let us suppose that a hungry dog has been taught, by the procedure indicated, to salivate upon the occurrence of a blinking light. And let us further suppose that provision is now made so that the dog himself can *turn on the light*. If given a convenient opportunity, will he do so? He *will,* repeatedly—thus indicating that a first-order conditioned stimulus can serve as a secondary reinforcer, not only in the sense of establishing higher-order salivary conditioning, but also in the sense of setting up *new habits*. If the blinking light can be turned on by nosing a "button" or pressing a lever with its paw, the dog will show a much more marked tendency to make such a response than if it produces no such stimulus. What is happening here is that the dog learns a new bit of behavior, not because that behavior produces (is rewarded by) food, but because it produces merely a sign, or *promise,* of food. How can this finding be explained?

9

In their study of salivary conditioning, Pavlov and his co-workers had been zealously objective and had meticulously limited their observations (or at least their scientific reports) to the action of the salivary gland, to the neglect of the dog-as-a-whole. As a result of conditioning experiments which were conducted and reproduced as motion pictures by Carl Zener (1937), it was demonstrated that a hungry dog, upon hearing or seeing a stimulus that signalizes food, not only salivates; the dog looks interested, hopeful, even "happy" and, if not physically restrained, will move bodily *toward* the place where the food is likely to be delivered.

From this and related observations it was justifiably inferred that, in a situation of the kind described, a conditioned stimulus not only makes the subject salivate: it also makes him *hopeful,* just as surely as a stimulus which has been associated with onset of pain makes a subject *fearful.* And if a fear-arousing stimulus elicits the two forms of *avoidance* behavior previously discussed, it might be surmised that a hope-arousing stimulus would be capable, likewise, of producing either of two forms of "approach" behavior, one of which has already been alluded to and which, in ordinary life, is exemplified by the family dog coming "when called." Just as an organism wishes to get *less* of a stimulus that makes it afraid (cf. Holt's concept of *abience,* 1931) and may do so by fleeing, so will an organism try to get *more* of a stimulus that arouses hope (Holt's *adience*) and may do so by going toward the source of that stimulus. Hence we emerge with an understanding of what has been called positive and negative *place* learning (spatial approach and avoidance).

But now let us suppose that the stimulation which precedes a rewarding state of affairs is *response-produced,* rather than environmentally produced. Let us suppose, that is to say, that a hungry animal makes a particular response, thereby stimulating itself in a characteristic manner, *and obtains food.* By principles already enunciated, we would expect the response-correlated stimulation to take on secondary reinforcement properties and that the subject, when again hungry, would now try to "get more" of *these* ("promising") stimuli. What would be the result? Since these "promising" stimuli are not located in space, the subject could not get more of them by going to any particular place. The only way to rouse or intensify them is for the subject to make or accentuate the *response* that has previously produced them! *And the tendency to make a particular response, in the presence of a particular drive or need, is what is ordinarily termed a "habit."*

According to Thorndike's classical statement of the Law of Effect, a habit consists of a strong "connection" between a particular stimulus or drive and a particular response. Although this connection was often said to be merely "functional" (or even "mathematical"), without necessarily implying anything about *neural* pathways, it was very natural to assume that the theory did presuppose the direct strengthening of neural connections. How otherwise was one to interpret the notion of a "connection"? The conception of habit just suggested is different in that it presupposes only that there is an improved or strengthened connection (a specifically neural connection rather than just a vaguely "functional" one) between certain end organs which are excited in specific ways by a given response *and the emotion of hope*. Hope is something which motivated organisms like to have (since it implies imminent drive reduction), just as fear is something they do *not* like to have (since it implies a threat of drive increase), so that we may legitimately infer that a motivated organism will show a strong tendency to make those responses which have, as one may say, a *hopeful* "feedback." The tendency to seek response-correlated stimulation which arouses hope is biologically useful in that it disposes a motivated organism to make responses which in the past have led to (or produced) satisfaction. Thus, as between the tendency noted earlier for living organisms to seek *external* stimulation which has been associated with reward and the tendency, just described, for them to seek *self-produced* stimulation which has been associated with reward, we have at least the rudiments of an explanation for goal-seeking behavior in general.

SYMMETRY AND SCOPE OF THE SYSTEM

Behavior, we thus discover, consists of two types of approach and avoidance tendencies. If an *independent stimulus* arouses fear, flight is likely to follow; whereas *response-correlated stimuli* which arouse fear produce inhibition. And if an independent stimulus arouses hope, approach will occur; whereas response-correlated stimuli which arouse hope produce response facilitation or "habit." And where response facilitation or response inhibition is concerned, it is not that a direct drive-behavior bond is either strengthened or weakened; instead it is a matter of the hope or fear that has gotten conditioned to the stimuli which are typically aroused by the occurrence of a particular pattern of action.

Stated most concisely, the thesis is that much of the adjustive, self-regulatory behavior of living organisms can be subsumed under four rubrics: the *avoidance* of places and the *inhibition* of responses which have been negatively (incrementally) reinforced and the *approach* to places and the *facilitation* of responses which have been positively (decrementally) reinforced. Thus the question of whether living organisms learn "responses" *or* "places" is resolved by the discovery that they are capable of and constantly manifest *both* forms of learning, which, however, involves one and the same set of principles: namely the conditioning of hopes and fears, under the impact of drive decrements and drive increments, to either independent or response-dependent stimuli. This way of thinking cuts the ground from under the controversy between "reinforcement theorists" and "field theorists" and provides the basis for a conceptual scheme of considerable generality and power (Mowrer, 1960a, Chap. 9).

This is still a two-factor, or two-process, conception of learning, but it differs from the preceding (second) version in certain important ways. The earlier version distinguished between sign learning and solution learning; the new version assumes that *all* learning is sign learning, or conditioning, and that solution learning (including inhibition) is a derivative or special case thereof. Wherein, then, is the theory still two-factored? It is still two-factored in that it assumes that there are two quite different forms of reinforcement: drive decrement (reward) and drive increment (punishment). In this respect the theory is congruent with common sense and with important aspects of many other psychological systems; but it deviates from the thesis of Hull (also favored for a time by Thorndike, 1931, 1932) that all reinforcement is decremental; and while agreeing with Tolman that all learning is sign learning, it is more "dynamic," less purely "cognitive." Finally, the new conception accepts "Pavlovian conditioning" as basic, but it goes considerably beyond Pavlov in stressing the essentially emotional (motivating and reinforcing) nature of condition responses; and it also holds that overt, instrumental behavior is much more complexly determined than Pavlov's (essentially reflexological) position assumed.

TWO-FACTOR THEORY DIAGRAMATICALLY PORTRAYED

Because it is not always easy to see precisely how the present conceptual scheme differs from the earlier "two-factor" positions, and because it is important that there be no ambiguity about this difference, this section will reproduce a discussion from an earlier study (Mowrer, 1956) which goes into this matter in some detail.

12

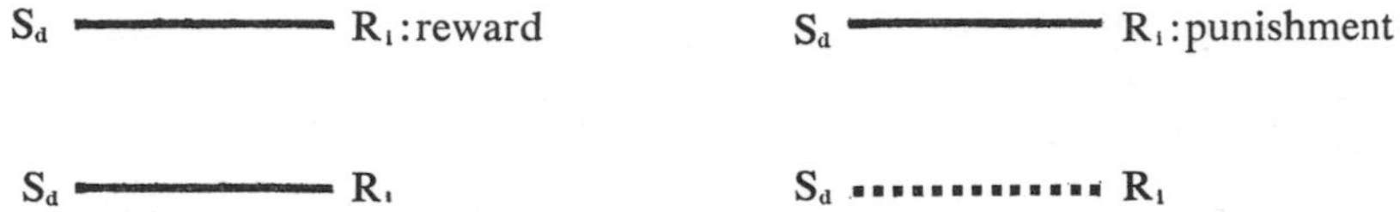

S_d ━━━━━ R_1: reward S_d ━━━━━ R_1: punishment

S_d ━━━━━ R_1 S_d ⋯⋯⋯ R_1

FIG. 1.—Schematic representation of the two halves, or aspects, of Thorndike's Law of Effect. It held, in essence, that if some drive stimulus S_d produces some instrumental (behavioral) response R_1, and if R_1 is then followed by reward, this S_d—R_1 sequence, or *bond,* will as a result be strengthened and that if such a stimulus-response sequence is followed by punishment, the bond will as a result be weakened.

The original, actually the *second,* version of two-factor learning theory now appears, in retrospect, as a sort of stepping stone, intermediate between monistic interpretations and the revised two-factor position here presented. The systematic relationships here involved may be summarized as follows:

Thorndike's Law of Effect is schematized in Figure 1 and the Pavlovian conception of conditioning is represented in Figure 2. Each alone, according to its exponents, was capable of accounting for the basic facts of learning; but others felt that both conceptions were necessary. Two-factor learning theory, as envisioned a decade ago, ac-

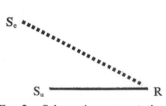

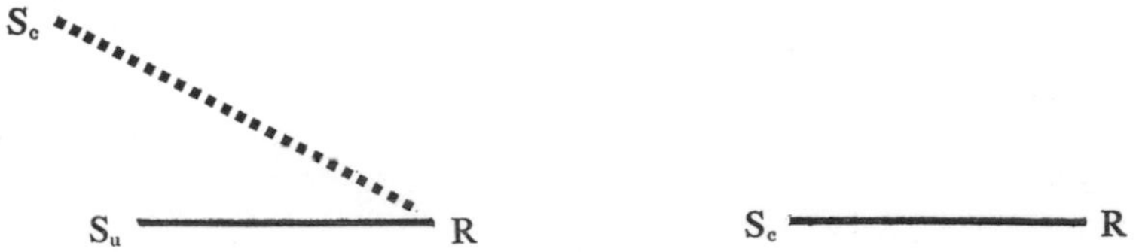

S_u ━━━━━ R S_c ━━━━━ R

FIG. 2.—Schematic representation of conditioning, as conceived by Pavlov. S_c is a stimulus which, initially, is not capable of eliciting response R, but which as a result of contiguous occurrence with S_u (above, at left), acquires this capacity (above right). The subscripts c and u are used to designate, respectively, what Pavlov termed the "conditioned" and the "unconditioned" stimulus.

cepted, essentially unmodified, the "first half" of the Law of Effect, which held that reward strengthens habit; but it departed from the Law of Effect in holding that punishment achieves its action, not by simply reversing the effects of reward, but by causing fears to become attached (conditioned) to stimulation associated with the occurrence of the punished response. This version of two-factor theory is shown in Figure 3. Here habit formation, or solution learning, is conceived essentially as Thorndike suggested; but punishment is seen in more complex terms. Instead of simply reversing the effect produced by past reward, pun-

13

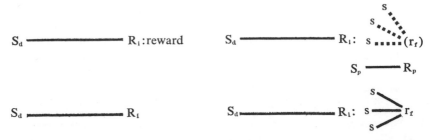

F<small>IG</small>. 3.—Schematic representation of the second version of two-factor learning theory. According to that formulation, habits were made by reward, as shown at the left, in essentially the way suggested by the Law of Effect. However, punishment was assumed to involve fear conditioning, as shown at right, with ensuing conflict and probably inhibition (see text).

ishment is here thought of as providing the basis for the conditioning of fear, which then produces conflict and, if the fear is strong enough, inhibition.[3]

The details of this interpretation of punishment are shown at the right in Figure 3. Here a problem situation or drive, S_d, produces an overt, instrumental response, R_i. R_i is followed by punishment, which is here represented as S_p. The punishment elicits a response R_p of which r_f, or fear, is a component. But when R_i occurs, it not only produces the extrinsic punishment, S_p; it also produces a number of other stimuli, s, s, s, which are inherently related to the occurrence of R_i. The result: a part of the reaction produced by S_p, namely fear, gets conditioned to these response-produced stimuli, s, s, s. Consequently, when S_d recurs the organism starts to perform R_i, the resulting stimuli "remind" the organism of the antecedent punishment, i.e., cue off r_f, which tends to inhibit R_i.

Two-factor learning theory, in its middle version, thus accepted Thorndike's conception of habit formation but derived the phenomenon of punishment from fear conditioning, rather than attributing it to a

3. Editor's note: Sheehan (1953a, 1958b) has developed a theory of stuttering which emphasizes this conflict nature of the problem with reference to the initial onset of stuttering and its perpetuation. He has used Miller's (1944) experimental studies of conflict as a frame of reference and has described stuttering as a double approach-avoidance conflict. Sheehan states, "For a stutterer both speech and silence have positive and negative features" (1958b, p. 125).

He views the primary symptoms of stuttering (repetitions and prolongations) as expressive of a basic conflict between the desire to speak and the desire to "hold back" from speaking. It is postulated that secondary symptoms are attempts to "filibuster" out of the conflict or "behavior symbolizing unconsciously the stutterer's attitude toward his listeners or toward life itself" (1958b, p. 129). (See Chap. 5, this volume.)

14

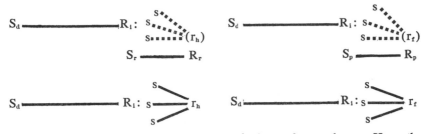

FIG. 4.—Schematic representation of revised two-factor theory. Here the changes produced in behavior by reward, as well as those produced by punishment, are derived from conditioning plus the feedback principle.

process which simply reversed the effects of past reward. As has been shown, this theory of punishment involves the same principles as have been found most satisfactory for explaining so-called avoidance learning. In both instances, fear becomes conditioned to stimuli, either external or response-produced, and the organism then makes whatever type of adjustment will most effectively eliminate these stimuli and reduce the attendant fear.

Current two-factor theory is diagrammed in Figure 4. Here it is assumed that habit formation is a matter of conditioning no less than is punishment. If a stimulus, S_d, produces a given response, R_i, and if R_i is followed by reward S_r, then it is assumed that part of the total response, R_r, which is produced by S_r, will become conditioned to the stimuli inherently connected with R_i. Here the conditionable component of R_r is r_h, the "hope" (secondary reinforcement) reaction; and it becomes connected to stimuli, s, s, s, just as fear does in the case of punishment. The result is that whenever R_i starts to occur, it is facilitated rather than inhibited.

THE NATURE OF UNLEARNING

Thorndike had a definite and simple, though probably mistaken, conception of unlearning. It was the process of "connection" weakening which resulted, as he believed, from punishment. And Pavlov saw unlearning as involving either of two processes: extinction *or* counterconditioning. A conditioned response, he found, will eventually stop occurring if it is not occasionally confirmed, or "reinforced," by the occurrence of the unconditioned stimulus. That is to say, if a promise (sign of reward) or a threat (sign of punishment) is repeated over and over again and not at least occasionally substantiated, or "made good," one would certainly expect the subject to stop responding: to continue indefinitely to react to no longer valid signs would not be biologically useful. And Pavlov repeatedly showed, by laboratory experiment, that extinction is a very definite and real phenomenon. Also, what is equally plausible, he showed that the response to a conditioned stimulus or sign can be modified by means of counterconditioning. Thus, if a sign has originally meant reward and if conditions are changed so that it now means punishment, we would expect the reaction produced thereby to change from hope (salivation, in Pavlov's experiments) to fear (Pavlov spoke of "defense reactions")—or vice versa. But as we have now seen, neither Thorndike's nor Pavlov's original formulation is entirely satisfactory; and having evolved a new and different conception of the learning process, we also must now come to grips with the problem of unlearning within this new system.

Revised two-factor learning theory assumes, as already indicated, that all learning, in the final analysis, is sign learning or conditioning—not conditioning in the sense of overt responses (or as mere "cognitions") but in the sense of positive and negative emotions, notably those of hope and fear, which then mediate and guide actual behavior (see also Mowrer, 1960b, Chaps. 2, 5). And since extinction and counterconditioning are recognized forms which unlearning takes where conditioned reactions are concerned, we here accept the assumption that these are the major (perhaps only) forms of unlearning. In the final analysis, extinction and counterconditioning may come down to the same thing, for a hope that is not confirmed is said to involve *disappointment* (which is a form of punishment) and a fear that is not confirmed provides *relief* (which is a form of reward). Therefore, it may be more precise to say that unlearning always involves counterconditioning, and that extinction is merely a species thereof. But, for the moment, this is not a pressing issue.

What is much more critical is the question of how one can accept a counterconditioning theory of unlearning and still be able to account for the manifest phenomenon of *conflict*. As already noted, one of the serious weaknesses of Thorndike's Law of Effect was that it had stimulus-response bonds being directly strengthened or weakened by reward and punishment, respectively, with no possibility of the subject ever experiencing frustration, confusion, or a sense of contradiction. And if we now assume that unlearning is simply a matter of the *sign* ("direction") of signs being changed, from positive to negative (hope to fear) or the reverse, there might seem to be here also equally little grounds for the experience of conscious conflict. A stimulus or situation would, presumably, be either "good, bad, or indifferent," but never "ambivalent." It would be strongly or mildly negative for the subject, strongly or mildly positive, or neutral; but it could not be positive and negative *at the same time,* and this, at least superficially, is the essence of conflict.

Although this problem cannot be said to have been fully solved, a promising possibility lies in the fact that any one response or any one situation involves a great number and variety of stimuli, some of which may, at a particular point in time, be conditioned to hope and others to fear. Thus, as the subject "attends" (Mowrer, 1960b) now to one, now to another set of stimuli, first one emotion (attitude) will predominate, then another. This could easily account for the back-and-forth vacillation sometimes seen in a conflicted organism and also explain why it is that such an organism is said to be of "two minds" about the situation (or action) in question. Only when all or at least a clear majority of the stimuli associated with a particular response or place become positive or negative does the individual become one-minded, unified, organized (Mowrer, 1960a, Chap. 11).

It seems, therefore, that the question of unlearning offers no serious difficulties to revised two-factor theory and helps clarify the form which the theory, of necessity, must take—although this treatment of conflict needs to be carefully checked against N. E. Miller's (1944) studies of approach-avoidance behavior. It is believed, however, that Miller's findings lend themselves rather nicely to reinterpretation along the lines suggested.

"PARADOXICAL" RESISTANCE TO EXTINCTION

It is important to say a word here about a paradox, sometimes known as the "Humphreys effect" (Skinner, 1938; Humphreys, 1939a, 1939b). If a stimulus is followed by reward, it acquires the capacity to arouse hope; if followed by punishment, the capacity to arouse fear; and if a stimulus which has been followed by either reward or punishment is now followed by "nothing," i.e., is not confirmed, it tends to lose the meaning it has previously possessed. Such at least would seem to be reasonable assumptions.

However, some twenty years ago it was discovered that if, during training, reinforcements occur *intermittently,* i.e., if reinforced trials are interspersed with nonreinforced trials, then in the *test* situation there will

17

be greater "resistance to extinction" than if reinforcement has occurred on each and every training trial. For example, if a hungry rat learns to press a little bar as a means of obtaining food, this "habit" will be more persistent after food has been discontinued if, during the training period, the subject has sometimes pressed the bar and received no food. From a common-sense point of view, this outcome does not seem very remarkable: persons, we observe, who have had a "hard time" are often more persevering, in the face of adversity, than are those who have "had it easy." But, in the light of learning-theory logic, the phenomenon has been puzzling.

On the assumption that hope (secondary reinforcement) is built up through the conjunction of a response (response-correlated stimulation) with reward and that hope is weakened by nonconfirmed occurrences of the response, then, for instance, fifty successive pairings of response and reward ought to produce more "habit strength" (hope) than fifty comparable rewarded occurrences of the response intermingled with, say, fifty nonrewarded (extinction) occurrences thereof. Consider the situation thus: if each rewarded occurrence of the response produces a certain increment of habit strength and if each nonrewarded occurrence produces a certain decrement, then any given number of successively rewarded occurrences of the response should "add up" to more habit strength than the same number of rewarded occurrences intermixed with any number of nonrewarded occurrences. That is to say, if each rewarded occurrence of the response is thought of as a + ("plus") and each nonrewarded occurrence as a − ("minus"), then any given number of +'s alone will sum to *more* than will the same number of +'s with −'s (however few) included.

Several different conjectures have been advanced to explain the Humphreys effect, of which the most satisfactory, until recently, was the so-called "discrimination hypothesis" (Mowrer and Jones, 1945; Bitterman, Feddersen, and Tyler, 1953). It goes as follows. When a subject has been intermittently reinforced during training, he continues to react, at least for a while, during the test period as if "nothing has happened," for the reason that response without reward is no novelty to him. That is to say he cannot, for a while, "tell the difference" between the conditions of intermittent reinforcement (which prevailed during training) and no reinforcement whatever (extinction); whereas if, during training, reward has been forthcoming on every trial, then the first nonrewarded (extinction) trial is different and the subject quickly senses that something is "wrong" and soon "stops work."

18

From a common-sense, intuitive standpoint, this interpretation seems very plausible; but its acceptance has been seen as something of a defeat for reinforcement theory in that the "discrimination hypothesis," as ordinarily formulated, is highly "cognitive" and seems to transcend ordinary reinforcement concepts (Woodworth, 1958). But thanks to a recent paper by Amsel (1958), it now seems that the Skinner-Humphreys effect was "paradoxical" because the whole process of extinction (unlearning) had been misconceived. As Amsel has been able to show, on both logical and empirical grounds, nonreinforcement is not a purely neutral (merely nonreinforcing) experience; it is, instead, a *frustration.* And what intermittent reinforcement during acquisition does, apparently, is not to produce a stronger habit (as increased resistance to extinction has been taken to mean) but rather to make extinction (*consistent* nonreward), when it finally comes, *less frustrating*—because the experience of nonreward has previously been interspersed with reward and its "sting" removed. In short, intermittent reinforcement seems to produce, not greater habit strength, but *diminished frustration effectiveness.*

Here, then, is an interpretation of the Humphreys effect which is in no way paradoxical but is, instead, fully in accordance with expanded reinforcement principles. They are expanded to the extent of assuming, not unreasonably surely, that the threat of punishment produces *fear,* that promise of a reward produces *hope,* and that a promise which has been made but not fulfilled produces *frustration* or *anger* which, along with fear, can serve to obliterate (counter-condition) hope. And from this it follows that when, during so-called intermittent reinforcement, frustration (due to nonreward) on one trial is shortly followed by reward on the next, then the reaction of frustration or anger on the nonrewarded trials gives way to *hope,* which is all that is needed to provide the basis for a highly parsimonious and "objective" explanation of the Humphreys effect.

Thus, the "discrimination hypothesis," which has usually been formulated in frankly cognitive terms, can be reformulated in a more systematic way: one which, to be sure, somewhat expands, but does not in the least impugn, our general "reinforcement" position.

UNIFYING POWER OF THE PRESENT THEORY

In addition to its incorporation of some of the basic thinking of Pavlov (1927) and its explanation of many of the phenomena which

19

particularly interested Thorndike (1932) revised two-factor theory (another name would serve as well, or better) is compatible with many of the premises of "field theory" and psychoanalysis. Here we may note especially the positive and negative "valences" which Lewin (1936) attributed to objects in psychological space and the positive and negative "cathexes" of which Freud (1920) often spoke. A positive "valence" or "cathexis," it seems, is simply that attribute ("hope" in our terms) which a stimulus acquires by virtue of its conjunction with important satisfactions; and a negative valence or cathexis, by the same token, is simply that attribute ("fear") which a stimulus acquires by virtue of its conjunction with discomfort or pain. Revised two-factor theory likewise is congruent with common-sense (and social-psychological) notions about positive and negative "interests" and "attitudes" (Allport, 1935; Thorndike, 1935).

II

EDWARD MURRAY

Social Learning, Personality Change,

and Psychotherapy

THERE ARE TWO THINGS I should like to accomplish in this presentation. First, I shall talk about some general ideas in learning theory, some basic principles that might be useful in understanding psychotherapy. Second, I should like to present some research on psychotherapy that I have done in collaboration with some co-workers, concentrating first on traditional individual psychotherapy, then on newer, more specialized kinds of psychotherapy, and finally on some other more general problems relating learning theory to psychotherapy.

LEARNING THEORY

First of all, why would one talk about learning concepts in connection with this field? One can conceive of the fields of mental health and psychopathology as the study of behavior patterns learned and exhibited

21

in the social context. Therefore, these fields can be viewed as involving problems in the acquisition and elimination of responses rather than problems of physical or medical disease. The disease concept has dominated those areas but the learning approach provides us with the alternative view that we are dealing with acquired behavior. In the future we will need a new vocabulary; we will have to drop terms like mental illness, neurosis, and psychopathology, and talk about the various kinds of behavior patterns that may be maladaptive. As a matter of fact, some writers have pointed out that the disease model has been holding back progress, but I do not wish to belabor this point.

If one is dealing then with patterns of social behavior, the principles of learning, to the extent that they are known, should apply to the original development of behavior problems and to the relearning involved in psychotherapy. There are many schools of learning, but my approach will be more or less eclectic. Within the learning theory group, if there is any one particular theory to which I owe a debt, it would be that of Dollard and Miller (1950).

I wish to go over a couple of key points that I will be using later on, starting with the Dollard and Miller analysis of learning. They specify four fundamental factors in the learning of a response: drive, cue, response, and reward. To give a very simple example of what is involved here: a drive would be something instigating action, for example, hunger, thirst, or fear on the physiological level or more complex drives on a social level. I will refer later to fear as a learned drive and to social drives, such as achievement. Hunger may motivate certain responses which, performed in the presence of a particular cue, lead to a reward; a reward is reduction of that original drive. I think human behavior is a little more complex than this but we always end up giving examples of people going to the refrigerator. A man is hungry, goes downstairs to the refrigerator, opens the door, gets out some salami and swiss cheese, and makes a sandwich. The drive here is obviously hunger, the cue is the refrigerator, the response is opening the door, and the reward is the food. Things can get more complicated. A friend of mine has purchased an expensive hunting dog that is supposed to point. The only problem is that this dog is so civilized, so domesticated, that all he has learned to do is point to the refrigerator, stand there with his tail out and paw pointing toward the refrigerator. He has learned to give that particular response to that particular cue.

The actual analysis of a given learning situation, whether in a laboratory or social situation, is more complex, and there are many processes involved. For example, a response is not always learned quickly just because it is followed by a reward. The reward may be less effective if it does not follow the response immediately. This particular principle involves the *gradient of reinforcement*. It is a temporal or a time gradient. If someone is to learn something, the reward should be given relatively quickly after the response, for the effectiveness of a reward drops off as time goes on. I will come back to this point later because I think it is significant with respect to some of the problems I shall discuss. A given response to a given cue may also be generalized to a different cue if it is similar to the original cue. If a person learns to respond to a tone of a given loudness and then a tone of a somewhat different loudness is produced, the person will respond, but not quite as frequently or with as great an amplitude. In a family situation, a boy may learn hostility toward his father, and this may be generalized later to people in positions of authority. So too, a response learned on the basis of reward can be eliminated through the process of *extinction*. Extinction occurs when a cue is presented and the individual performs the response, but nothing happens, no reward is given. Eventually, the response will stop occurring. After a response is extinguished it can recur through a process called *spontaneous recovery*. An example will clarify this. Suppose that you are trying to open a door and suddenly it is stuck. You keep trying and you still cannot get it open so finally you give up. The next day you know that it is still stuck but you try anyway, this response comes back; in other words extinction is not an absolute thing. It can wear off, so to speak.

Until World War II, most learning psychologists concentrated on the kinds of processes I have just mentioned, but more recently there has been a great deal of interest in the so-called *higher mental processes* involved in learning. The literature sometimes gives the impression that learning involves the relationship between an external stimulus and an overt observable response. But, as a matter of fact, most social learning involves some kind of verbalization whether it is overt or covert; it may involve internal symbolic processes which cannot be observed but which are the mediating processes important in all social learning. Dollard and Miller (1950) present a very detailed analysis of this. For example, without a verbal response, how would you ever learn to tell that five dimes and a fifty cent piece are the same in value? They look quite different yet they mean the same thing. The meaning is given by a mediating verbal response that these both add up to fifty cents worth of money. The higher mental processes are extremely important in understanding not only pathological behavior, but all behavior on the human level.

One other process studied by learning theorists and particularly important in understanding neurosis and psychotherapy is the idea of a *learned drive*. Suppose it was noted that an experimental animal or a human being showed a fear reaction to a given stimulus. John Watson discovered many years ago that an infant would respond with intense fear if a loud sound was produced suddenly behind its head. This is unlearned; it just seems to happen with babies. It can become a learned response by associating a previously neutral stimulus with this unconditioned stimulus. For example, one can have a light go on just before this loud noise. After several pairings, the light by itself will elicit the fear response. This is called a learned fear or anxiety reaction. Fear seems to have motivating properties because once aroused it is a painful, uncomfortable psychophysiological state. A person would want to get rid of it. How can he? People learn various kinds of responses to reduce anxiety or fear. Since one definition of drive is "strong stimuli which impel action," fear has been called a learned drive.

Most symptoms of psychopathology may be viewed as anxiety-reducing responses. A phobia is an example of such a symptom. A person may be afraid of a given area and keeps avoiding it; there is something about this particular area that arouses anxiety. Such a phobia may be viewed as a simple avoidance phenomenon. Sometimes it is more complicated. Dollard and Miller (1950) describe the case of a girl who had a phobic reaction among other problems. She retained a behavior pattern from her lower-class youth of going out on the streets and picking up men. After her marriage to a middle-class man, she stopped this pattern of behavior. However, the marriage was going badly, and every once in a while she would have an urge to go out and pick up a man. When this happened it made her quite anxious, as one might well imagine, because her marriage was at stake. Two things happened: one was that the thoughts involved here—the sexual thoughts—were repressed. She no longer realized why she had an urge to take a walk. The verbal mediating responses, such as "I have certain needs," were eliminated. Why? Because they caused a great deal of anxiety when they were evoked. In dynamic terminology they were repressed; in learning terms they were inhibited. At the same time, the fear reaction was avoided by not going out on the streets. This left her in a peculiar position; she had a fear of going out on the streets but could not tell you why. Here is a classical neurotic picture in which the person has a

24

symptom, obviously highly motivated, but can give no explanation of it. By the way, some of this might be related to Mowrer's concept (1965b) that the central problem in personality disturbance is guilt that is realistic. It is not likely that therapy in her case would consist of removing her inhibition and encouraging her toward sexual freedom. Obviously her major problem could be stated in terms of the difficulties she was having in the marital relationship with her husband. Probably one of the worst things to do would be to remove her inhibitions about going out indiscriminately with men, for this would entirely disrupt her marital situation. I think there is a difference between the way I have phrased the problem and the way Mowrer might, but there is also a similarity.

I might make a few more comments about anxiety. Anxiety or fear can be viewed as a psychophysiological reaction to danger which may sometimes be adaptive and sometimes not. In many of the early learning studies fear was aroused by some kind of a physical stimulus: an electric shock, a blast of air on the face of a cat, and other painful stimuli of a physical sort. This has given many people the idea that the kind of fear studied by learning theorists is a very physical kind of fear. In fact, recent data suggests that the origin of many fears is social rather than physical. For example, one can produce fear reactions in animals by placing them in strange, startling situations. This can be seen in the child, too. An infant or child, who, let us say at the age of one, is brought into a new situation, will start crying. A child of eight months, when introduced to a stranger, may show extreme anxiety. The studies by Harlow, in which monkeys learn to cling to inanimate objects made to look somewhat like their monkey mothers, suggest that when monkeys are in a strange situation or simply in open field, they show signs of panic. This panic seems to be related to social contact; these fears and anxieties tend to be reduced when the monkey can cling to his surrogate mother. When a child is frightened he clings to his mother, and the reduction in anxiety is visible.

A number of important factors are involved in these fears. There is a critical period during the first few months when the monkey learns to cling to the mother to reduce anxiety. The maternal deprivation studies show that if a child does not learn to make this kind of an anxiety-reducing attachment to the mother during the first year of life, later on he may not make any social attachments at all. Therefore, anxiety is very closely tied up with social relationships. I think this is extremely important and I am convinced that this is a central phenomenon in all of psychopathology. For example, a person who has not learned to seek

25

others when anxious and to use other people for reducing his anxieties may become asocial or antisocial. On the other hand, some people are unable to learn any other way of dealing with anxiety except by a clinging, dependent kind of relationship with other people. In some family situations children learn that this affectionate response on the part of others, which seems to reduce anxiety, is made contingent upon the child doing various kinds of things, such as achieving high marks in school and so on. The administration of this kind of anxiety-reducing social experience facilitates social living.

One further aspect in the case of the woman with street-walking tendencies cited by Dollard and Miller may illustrate another principle involved in neurosis. There is a *conflict*. In her case there is a sex-anxiety conflict. The woman had sexual impulses which were blocked by anxiety. One way to describe this is to call the sexual motivation an approach tendency and the anxiety an avoidance tendency. As the approach tendency motivated responses of going out and walking down the street, the anxiety motivated responses of avoiding walking down the street. This kind of approach-avoidance conflict may be very important in psychopathology; not just sex anxiety but many other kinds of conflict such as aggression anxiety or achievement anxiety are also significant.

Miller (1944) has a theory on this kind of conflict. Figure 5, a graphic representation of conflict theory, is a model with two dimensions: (1) nearness to the goal, and (2) strength of behavior tendency. The tendency to go toward the goal varies and may be strong or weak. One of the propositions of the theory is that the closer you get to a given goal, the stronger the tendency to go toward the goal becomes. This is called the goal gradient and has been shown in laboratory experiments. For example, an animal running down the alley to get food at the end of it will run faster as he gets closer to the goal. When I was living in Virginia a friend of mind had to go to Texas for two months to receive some special army training. He was separated from his wife during this time and at the end of it, driving home, he noticed that his speed changed as he went from state to state. As he was going through Louisiana his speed was under the limit, but I guess he really flew through the last part of Virginia. Likewise a tendency to avoid a goal varies from weak to strong. If a laboratory animal is shocked at a distinctive point in an alley, it will tend to have a stronger avoidance reaction the nearer it is to the source of shock.

These approach and avoidance tendencies have been investigated in a

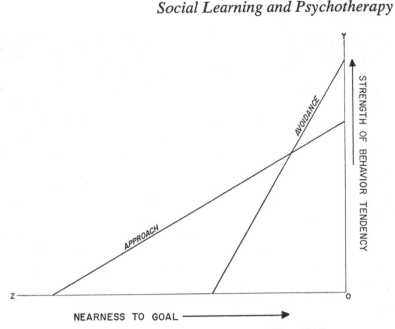

Fɪɢ. 5.—Miller's Model of Conflict (after Miller, 1944).

series of laboratory studies by Miller (1944). Miller measured the strength of approach and avoidance tendencies in laboratory rats that were attached by harnesses and cords to a scale that registered the strength of the animal's pull. After initial training the animals were restrained at different points as they were approaching or running away. In approaching the rats would pull with a greater force toward the food as they came closer to it. With reference to the avoidance tendency, the animals would pull away harder the nearer they were to the point of shock.

One other major assumption in this theory is that the approach gradient is flatter than the avoidance gradient, as shown in Figure 5. Stating it another way, the avoidance gradient tends to be steeper and falls off more rapidly than the approach gradient. This is why there is conflict. If they were both exactly the same steepness nothing would happen. It is only in the particular kind of situation where the strength of approach and avoidance tendencies differ that there is a conflict situation. If a laboratory animal is trained to run down a runway to get food and then shocked at the goal, he is in a conflict. After a few trials the

27

animal will start approaching the goal; he will get about half-way, and then start moving back and forth, or oscillating. This point is indicated in Figure 5 by the gradients' intersection.

The point of conflict depends on the strengths of the approach and avoidance gradients. For example, if the animal is given a very strong shock, the avoidance gradient is elevated. If given a very small shock, the avoidance gradient might be very low. In this latter case, he might make it all the way to the goal although acting a little nervous just as he approached it. It is only when these things are balanced that there is strong conflict: where the avoidance is just strong enough to inhibit the response but not strong enough to keep him out of the entire situation. There are some obvious relationships between this kind of theoretical analysis and various kinds of symptoms including stuttering. I will mention a few of these. Later, in addition, other authors in this volume comment specifically on conflict theory and stuttering.

Traditional Psychotherapy

I should like now to summarize a series of studies in which we attempted to take some of these ideas of learning and apply them to traditional psychotherapy, including the various kinds of therapy done by analysts, both Freudian and neo-Freudian, by Rogerians, by eclectics, and by many others. I am referring to the kind of therapy in which a patient comes in and talks to the therapist for "x" number of hours and at the end we think maybe something has happened.

I shall refer to some work previously summarized (Murray, 1964). A series of studies reported there utilized the method of content analysis as one way of studying psychotherapy. In recent years there has been a great deal of interest in tape recording psychotherapy sessions, and I was lucky enough to have access to a number of people who were doing psychotherapy and who were interested in this approach. Typically, we would get tape recordings of psychotherapy sessions, have them transcribed into a script, and then study the script. Sometimes the actual tape recordings are the basis of various content ratings.

The particular content analysis study in which I was interested revolved around categories of motivation, anxiety, and conflict. For example, there were categories of independence, dependence, affection, and sexual striving; fears in the sexual area, fears in the achievement area, fears of independence, and so forth. There were special categories for

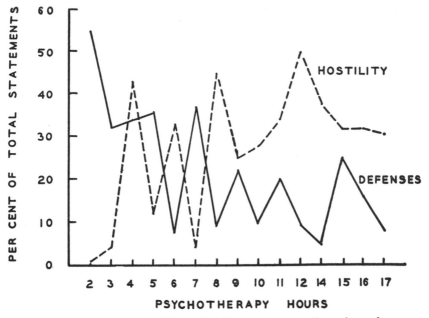

Fig. 6.—Percentage of hostility and defense statements throughout therapy—young college graduate (after Murray, 1954).

symptoms and defenses. Other categories were used to describe various aspects of the therapist's behavior. Typically, what we did was to take the flow of the patient's speech and divide it into simple sentences which we called meaning units. Then we would rate each one of these sentences or sequences of sentences as being indicative of a sexual problem or as being aggressive, hostile, defensive, and so forth. We found that we achieved fairly adequate reliability using trained judges. The total number of sentences for an hour was determined and the percentage in each category calculated. These are the basic data.

Figure 6 shows the results of a content analysis of a single case. The ordinate carries the percentage of total statements in a given category, the abscissa the hours in therapy. This is a psychotherapy case that extended over 17 sessions. The first hour was eliminated because it was a formal history-taking, and hour 13 is also missing. This particular case was a young college student who had a fear of dying in his sleep, as well as a number of physical complaints. Like many students, he also had all kinds of philosophical interests. He was a very passive, unaggressive individual, at least on the surface, and when he came in he exhibited no hostility at all. The therapy was analytically oriented and permissive.

The first hour of therapy was dominated by defensive statements (Fig. 6, solid black line). In his case, there were two types of defenses involved: one was intellectual preoccupations and the other physical complaints. He would come in and give a long description of his physical symptoms or an intellectual discourse consisting of rambling philosophical discussions, quite interesting, but with little relationship to his particular life problems. Why would a person come in and spend all this time talking about abstract things or physical complaints? One possibility—and this is our theory—is that this behavior was motivated by anxiety; the person was afraid to discuss certain subjects. There are many things that people are afraid to talk about. When a person first enters therapy this kind of fear is strong. All through therapy, because of the permissiveness of the therapist, I think there is a reduction in this anxiety; there is a decrease in the verbalizations of defenses over time. The defenses are assumed to be motivated by anxiety. When the anxiety is reduced the defenses also drop out.

The anxiety was also inhibiting the other arm of the conflict, and in this case it seemed to be hostility. Note the percentage of hostile statements this individual did express eventually.

Figure 6 should be examined carefully because it illustrates a number of things. The up-and-down, crisscross character of the lines looks very much like what a rat exhibits in the experimental alley and what is called conflict oscillation. After a few hours of therapy, the defensive statements decrease and the patient begins exhibiting hostility; however, the next hour the defenses reappear. The following hour he comes in with more problems involving hostility, but the defenses return once again. A seesaw effect characterizes this middle phase of therapy. Finally, he gets to the point where the expression of hostile feelings dominates the sessions for quite some time. Anxiety is not simply eliminated, but there is vacillation which gradually diminishes. I will now turn to some other material that shows even more dramatic examples of this.

The next case is a young schizophrenic girl who was treated by John Rosen.[1] The girl had a number of symptoms; there was some very vague

1. Rosen is a psychoanalyst who has specialized for many years in the treatment of psychotic individuals. He uses his own particular theoretical approach, which he calls direct analysis, interpreting the patient's behavior in very primitive Freudian terms. For example, a patient will show some concern about his mother

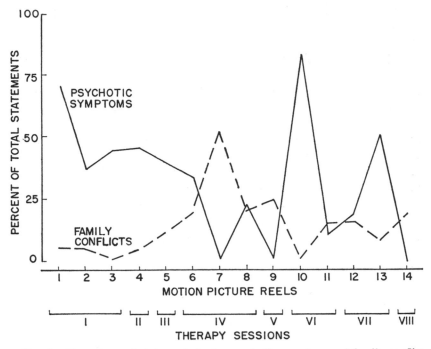

Fig. 7.—Percentage of statements in the psychotic symptom and family conflict categories—Rosen's Case A (after Murray, 1962).

religiosity, and there was a great deal of concern about sexual identity and a number of other things. These symptoms were at odds with a category called family conflicts. This is a very young immigrant girl. Her family were immigrants, and in many ways she was solving some of the classical problems of the second generation of Americans. She had many concerns about her parents, conflicts with them, a lot of it revolving around independence. She was trying to break away from home but could not. In a sense she was in an insoluble conflict.

Movies were made of the therapy sessions and transcripts were taken from the sound tracks. Figure 7 shows that therapy was initially dominated by discussions of psychotic symptoms. This would be analogous to the defenses in the case of the neurotic. Family conflicts were not

and John Rosen will say, "Ah, your mother's milk was no good, my milk is good; trust me and not your mother." This is one of the milder kinds of interpretations that he gives.

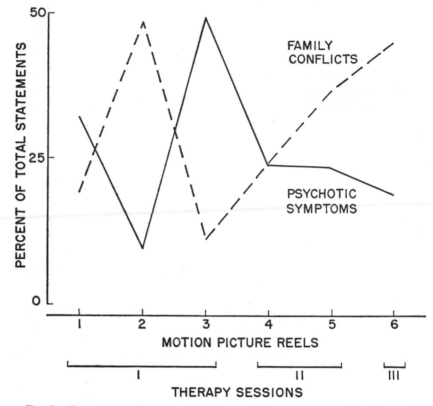

FIG. 8.—Percentage of statements in the psychotic symptom and family conflict categories—Rosen's Case B (after Murray, 1962).

immediately discussed—they slowly came to dominate the discussion, however, and the peak on reel 7 is what I think most psychotherapists would call a productive hour, an hour when a great deal of important material of dynamic significance was discussed. But as can be seen, the statements concerning family conflict fell off again. Something very dramatic happened between sessions 4 and 6. The patient was on a home visit, and these visits are important in therapy. They can produce disastrous results, in terms of the progress the patient is making. Eventually the patient has to be able to tolerate this, but sending a patient back to the home environment may undo all that the therapist has accomplished up to that point. The interesting thing here is that when she came

32

back from the weekend with her parents, she was obviously upset. What did she talk about, what was she exhibiting? Not the family conflicts category. Now if the family conflicts category represented one concern and the psychotic symptoms another, then when she came back from this difficult weekend with her parents she should have exhibited a lot of interest in the family conflicts. Instead, she was completely preoccupied with various delusional ideas. I think that this demonstrates the dynamic relationship between the psychotic symptom category and the anxiety. It shows that psychotic symptoms operate as a defense too.

I might mention briefly Figure 8, which shows another case treated by Rosen in which the same categories are used and in which the same kind of relationship is shown. Here there is an inverse relationship between psychotic symptoms and family conflicts.

Anxiety Reduction

Another observation of interest is the initial reduction in anxiety which is very typical of almost any kind of therapy. It has been called a placebo effect, and sugar pills will produce it under the right conditions. However, it may not have any relation to the long-range welfare of the individual. What I think it has to do with is initial contact, almost like the baby monkey touching the surrogate mother. After the initial anxiety-reduction the patient can talk about conflict areas, but this conflicting material raises more anxiety and he gets into an oscillating period of feeling more and then less comfortable. When he feels uncomfortable, when the anxiety is higher, there is one maneuver after another to get away from the anxiety-producing material. This may be called a negative therapeutic effect. After going into a topic and showing some real progress the individual then reverts to the old symptoms. However, this paradox can be explained in terms of conflict theory. If a person makes progress along a conflict dimension, like the one shown in Figure 5, as he gets past the point of conflict, anxiety increases. In a sense, the person scares himself and has to move back.

Another event that may take place is known as displacement. There are several examples of this, but one is shown in Figure 9. This is from the case of the college student mentioned earlier. Shown here is the hostility category (see Figure 6) now broken down into "targets" or people toward whom the hostility is expressed. The first big burst of hostility by this young college student is toward his mother. I will not engage in a complicated explanation. I will just say that most of his problems revolved around his mother and that was his basic complaint.

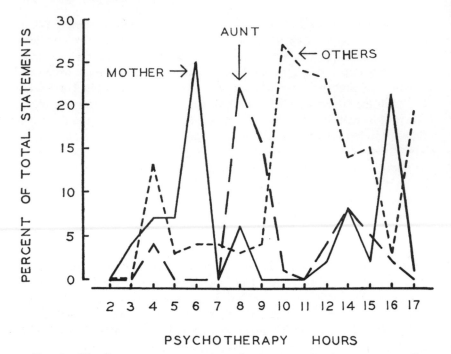

FIG. 9.—Hostile statements toward mother, aunt, and others—young college graduate (after Murray, 1954).

The next expression of hostility was toward his aunt, who also lived with them and created some problems too, but probably not as many as the mother. She served as a kind of scapegoat or displacement object for the hostility. During the middle of therapy, the hostility was expressed in a very generalized way to other, relatively insignificant people in the student's life. In other words, he kept moving away from the real source of the problem. It was only toward the end of therapy that he returned to the mother and, when he did return, the hostility expressed was much stronger and about much more significant things.

Why does therapeutic progress take place at all? My explanation is that anxiety extinction has taken place. But how does one know this has happened? Also, if anxiety extinction has taken place, should there not be a constant reduction in the level of tension exhibited by the person? This is not necessarily true, because the person may be going into deeper conflicts.

34

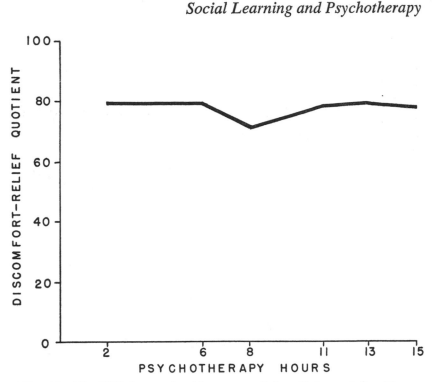

Fɪɢ. 10.—The DRQ in sample of hours—marital conflict case (after Murray, Auld, and White, 1954).

Let me illustrate by making reference to a different measure used in another case. This concerns a middle-aged married woman who had a number of problems. The Discomfort Relief Quotient, shown in Figure 10, is a measure devised by Dollard and Mowrer (1947). It involves counting the number of tense or discomfort words and the number of pleasurable or comfortable words, relief words, then calculating the ratio between the two groups of words. The significant thing shown in Figure 10 is that there is no essential change in this quotient throughout therapy. This is rather startling because the therapist involved in the case, as well as the supervisor, felt very strongly that a great deal of therapeutic progress had been made. Yet there is no drop in the Discomfort Relief Quotient. Why was this happening? One reason is that although progress occurred, it occurred through a substitution of one conflict area for another as the patient went along.

I went back to the original data in the case and applied the content

35

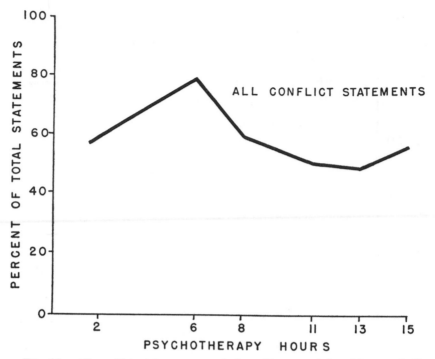

FIG. 11.—All conflict statements—marital conflict case (after Murray, Auld, and White, 1954).

analysis method. Figure 11 shows the sum of all of the various kinds of conflicts the person discussed. As with the Discomfort Relief Quotient there is no essential change. In other words, conflicting materials are being discussed all during the therapy.

The content, however, was changing, as shown in Figure 12. Initially the patient talked mainly about conflicts concerned with her mother and her daughter. While these were important, they did not seem to be the focal problem, at least they were not the only problem. As time went by statements about mother-daughter conflicts decreased and statements about conflicts with her husband increased. Furthermore, Figure 13 shows that the material about the husband shifted from a very general hostility conflict to a conflict about their sexual adjustment.

One can argue about which was the basic conflict and which was not, but I think most people would agree that this represents some shift

36

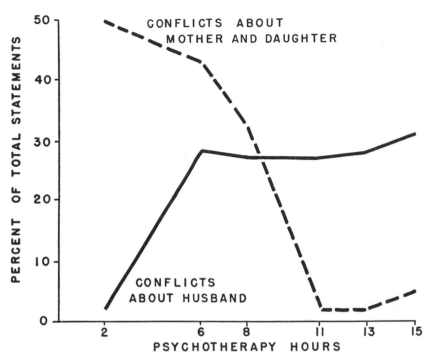

Fig. 12.—Conflicts about mother and daughter *versus* conflicts about husband—marital conflict case (after Murray, Auld, and White, 1954).

toward more significant material. More important is the fact that therapeutic change can occur even though the overall tension stays high. Therefore, one would not necessarily expect a simple steady reduction in anxiety during psychotherapy.

I am suggesting here that as anxiety extinction involving one conflict occurs, the person goes on to another conflict, possibly a more important one. This process is then a series of successive extinction procedures.

But is it really extinction? In order to answer this, I think it necessary to use a different kind of measure and actually get at this psychophysiological reaction called anxiety. This was done by a colleague of mine, James Dittes (1957), using the galvanic skin response. The psychotherapy case studied was a young man who had, among other difficulties, a sexual problem. He found it difficult to talk about sexual matters, but

37

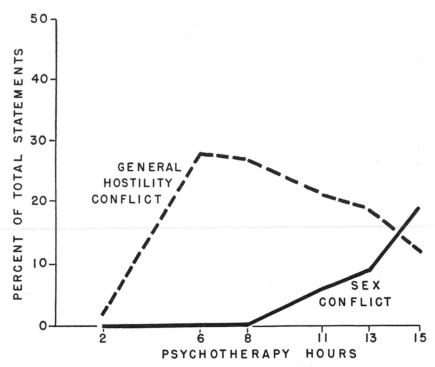

FIG. 13.—Hostility conflict *versus* sexual conflict—marital conflict case (after Murray, Auld, and White, 1954).

not about sex in general. He had trouble talking about the "embarrassing" aspects of sex. Embarrassing sexual material was rated by judges listening to tapes of the therapy hours. A continuous record was made of the patient's galvanic skin responses. Figure 14 shows that there was a decrease over a number of interviews in the percentage of times that he reacted to embarrassing sexual statements with this physiological anxiety reaction. There is also an up-and-down quality to this, quite typical of extinction curves. This supports the theory that anxiety extinction is a central phenomenon in psychotherapy.

THE ROLE OF THE THERAPIST

So far I have dealt with anxiety and conflict in the early stages of traditional psychotherapy and how anxiety extinction may take place.

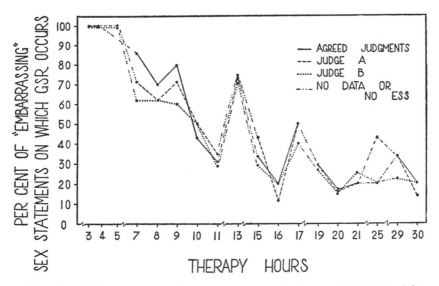

FIG. 14.—GSR to embarrassing sex statements during psychotherapy (after Dittes, 1957).

Also, up to now I have been discussing therapy as if the patient were sitting in a vacuum with no one else in the room. I have made very little reference to what the therapist does.

When one considers what the therapist does, and what he does that can be studied, it is at once obvious that he responds verbally to some of the things the patient says. Whether or not the verbal reactions of the therapist have some effect on what the patient says has been one area of investigation. For example, on a global level, there is a study by Glad (1959), who surveyed patients in therapy with therapists of different theoretical persuasions—Freudians, Rankians, Sullivanians, Rogerians, and others. He found that after therapy the patients spoke about their problems in terms of the theoretical emphasis of their particular therapist. For example, the patients who went to Freudian therapists would talk about their sexual and aggressive problems; those who went to Rogerian therapists talked about their problems in terms of emotional understanding, self-growth, and so on; those who went to Sullivanian therapists spoke about their problems in interpersonal relations; and those who saw Rankians spoke about autonomy. What this means, I think, is that the different problems of people can be described in various

39

theoretical terms. What is actually happening in therapy is that these problems get phrased in slightly different ways, and I think it is possible to translate them from one language system to another.

One other related study by Rosenthal (1955) indicated that successful patients tended to adopt the therapist's moral values. This suggests an identification with the therapist and also suggests that somehow the therapist, although he is supposed to be neutral and impassive, is communicating his value system.

Other studies show that therapists tend to select for treatment patients more similar to themselves. For example, I have been in many intake conferences at various mental health facilities in which there are more patients than therapists. Very often it is kind of a fishing game in which someone present will say, "Well, here is a person with this kind of problem, this kind of background. Who wants him?" Then someone says, "Oh, I would like that one." There is a pecking order in this; the more experienced, mature therapist tends to get patients who have more education, are more verbal, come from a higher socio-economic group, and so forth. Therapists, generally speaking, have been shown to reward upward socio-mobility, upward striving, and to be very upset if the patient shows downward mobility. I am not saying that therapists are wrong about this necessarily, but just that they do have views and values and that these do get across to the patient.

There has been an emphasis in traditional psychotherapy on the therapist not projecting his views into the therapy situation. Since our studies reveal evidence that the therapist does project his views, there has been a great deal of interest in how this might occur. One mechanism that has been suggested is the so-called Greenspoon effect. This refers to a study (Greenspoon, 1955) in which people were asked to simply sit in a room and say words, any words that came into their minds. The experimenter sat behind them and every time the person mentioned a plural noun, the experimenter said "un-hum." The incidence of plural nouns increased in frequency.

By the way, "un-hum" is one of the most frequently heard sounds in psychotherapy. Krasner (1961) has reviewed this area and found that verbs or nouns or whatever verbal class can be reinforced and their occurrence increased. Swiveling in the chair can be a reinforcing event. In one study, whenever a schizophrenic said something that had any kind of feeling the therapist would swing around in his chair and look at him. This seemed to be reinforcing. I do not want to get into the question of awareness. I think many of these things are quite conscious.

40

Some years ago I became interested in the problem and the question of whether it is possible for a therapist not to influence a patient. There is a therapist, Carl Rogers, who claims to be non-directive. I did a study on a case report which was published in Rogers' book, *Counseling and Psychotherapy* (1942), to see what the relationship was between therapist behavior and patient verbalizations.

My procedure was to score the patient's verbalization using the content categories I mentioned previously. The categories in this case included defenses and independence-dependence conflicts. First, I simply counted the number of times the therapist reacted to different content areas. Secondly, certain categories were scored as rewarded or punished by the therapist, and all I mean by this is that he said something positive or negative after a statement by the patient. These responses by the therapist were rated by a number of people and there was good agreement as to whether they were responses expressing approval or disapproval, or as I call them here, rewarded or punished. Some of the rewards were quite obvious things like "good," "great," and so forth. Punishing responses by the therapist were not punitive to the person in a humiliating sense, but punishing in the sense of being disapproving of the particular things the person was talking about. For example, at one time he said something like, "Well the real question is whether you can look at yourself or just look at some kind of an intellectualized version of yourself." This had a punitive effect on the person's subsequent intellectualizing. The therapist also said things like, "Well, it seems to me the choice is between going ahead or going back." Who in American society wants to go back? So he stopped talking about going back.

The results are given in Figure 15. I grouped all of the categories to which the therapist responded in a rewarding way, and it can be seen that these increased throughout the course of the therapy. I grouped all the punished categories, and these decreased.

Since the Greenspoon effect was discovered, it has become quite an important area of psychotherapy research. Some people have come to the conclusion that verbal reinforcement is a magical way of changing behavior, that all one has to do, essentially, is to decide what the patient is to be like and then sit there and reward him. The implication seems to be that behavior can be changed very radically just by saying "un-hum" at the right time. Unfortunately, I don't think it is that simple, and more and more data supports my position.

One study done at Indiana University by Kenneth Heller (1963) utilized a laboratory situation which was set up to be an analogue of

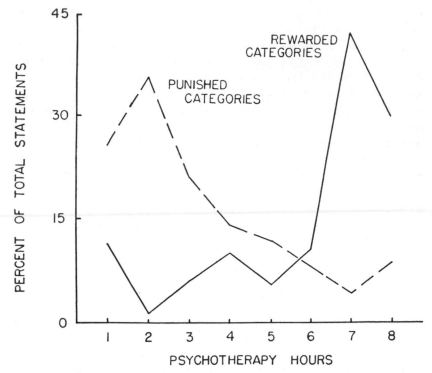

FIG. 15.—Categories approved or disapproved by the therapist—non-directive case (after Murray, 1956).

psychotherapy. Subjects were brought into a laboratory and asked to speak about anything that came into their minds. There was a programmed tape recorder to give approval at various intervals. The subject was just talking into a microphone and he thought somebody was in the other room listening, but it was just a tape recorder. He would hear, "Good, let's hear more of that," and so forth. Theoretically, this should increase the verbal productivity. Actually, it was too mechanical and it increased productivity only initially, but then productivity decreased. The conclusion I drew from this study was that a person does not want simple approval in a mechanical way but he wants discriminating approval. People seem to want approval from someone who is making a distinction between whether behavior is really adequate or not. Subjects, by the way, did not like this experiment; they did not like the constant approval. They even preferred a tape that was punishing or disapproving as well as approving.

If verbal reinforcement doesn't necessarily change behavior, what else is involved? First, I think it can be deduced from learning theory that a reward is only meaningful in connection with a drive or motive of some kind. I think verbal reinforcement is based on some kind of social motive. For example, there is one study by Sapolsky (1960) showing that verbal reinforcement, or the effectiveness of verbal reinforcement, depends on the personality compatibility between the therapist and the subject. This was an experimental study in which therapists or people acting as verbal reinforcers and subjects were given a personality test and then matched in various ways. Some of them were put together in congenial pairs, others in antagonistic pairs. It was found that the verbal conditioning procedure was much more effective when the pairs were compatible, but when they were incompatible it was not very effective at all. There is some evidence that in successful therapy patients end up liking and respecting their therapists. This suggests that the way to change someone's attitude, or to change someone's opinion about something, is to have information given to him by someone for whom he has respect. I have come to the conclusion that verbal reinforcement in psychotherapy is a secondary phenomenon, that its success is dependent upon the relationship between therapist and patient.

Another way of studying the therapeutic relationship is simply to see what happens during therapy in terms of the patient talking about the therapist. This is a rough measure of a complex matter, but it shows a certain interesting relationship. The relevant content category is shown in Figure 16. This category includes everything that was said about the therapist in a group of therapy cases, varying in length. There is an increase in statements about the therapist in every case. This suggests that there is an increase in positive and negative feelings, an increase in anxiety, in hostility, sexual feelings, affection, and so forth. The conclusion I draw from these data is that what develops is a complex human relationship with many feelings—positive, negative, and neutral.

I was also very much interested in discovering whether the therapist could reinforce transference material; that is, is this just something that the therapist encourages and therefore an effect of verbal reinforcement? Earlier I mentioned several of the cases treated by Rosen. Figure 17 shows the material connected with the case of the eighteen-year-old schizophrenic girl (Case A). There is a sharp, dramatic increase near the end of therapy. The other case, a man about forty years old and

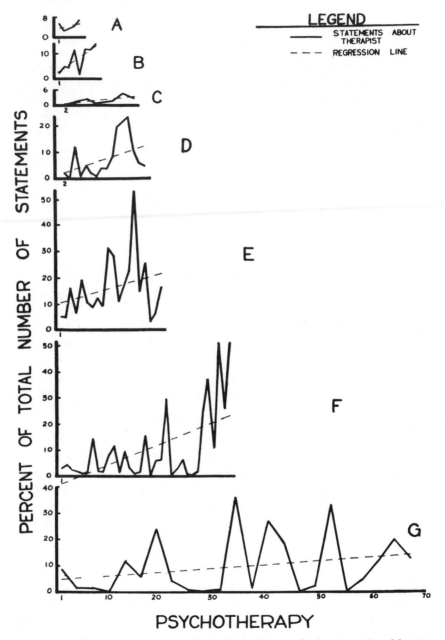

FIG. 16.—Statements about the therapist during psychotherapy (after Murray, 1956).

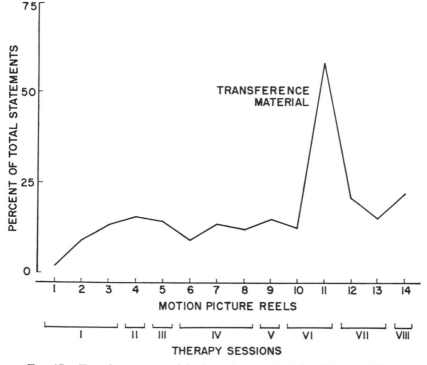

FIG. 17.—Transference material—Rosen's Case A (after Murray, 1964).

quite paranoid (Case B), is shown in Figure 18. This case also shows an increase but not so great. Note that the measurement units are different in Figures 17 and 18. In Figure 18 the increase in transference material is very small. As a matter of fact, Rosen had a great deal of trouble in establishing a relationship with this man. He had a much easier time with the eighteen-year-old girl. This might be related to Rosen's activity as shown in Table 1. In this table the percentage of patient's statements to which the therapist reacted, in three different categories, are given. The first thing to notice is that he is responding more to the transference material than to anything else. However, in Case B he is responding to an even greater degree to the transference material but, as I noted above, getting nowhere. This becomes even clearer in Table 2, which shows the same thing, except here I have divided the statements into those that are very active statements, conveying a good deal of information and mean-

45

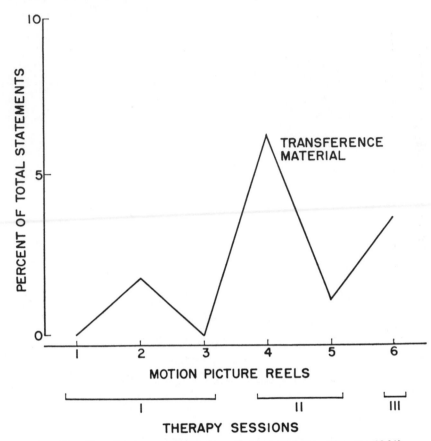

FIG. 18.—Transference material—Rosen's Case B (after Murray, 1964).

ing, and those that are minimal statements, just the "un-hum" and "yes" types. Rosen is trying even harder here, as evidenced by the more active responses to transference material. In conclusion, what seems to be happening is that Rosen was reacting to transference material more frequently than to other types of material, which is one reason he is getting an increase. But in Case B, where he was reacting very strongly with all kinds of reinforcement, he could not get an increase of any great magnitude. My clinical impression is that his relationship with the girl was a much more positive one than with the man. This confirms my

TABLE 1

THERAPIST REACTION TO PATIENT
CONTENT CATEGORIES

Patient Content Categories	Percentage of Patient Statements to which Therapist Reacted	
	Case A	Case B
Psychotic symptoms	19	34
Family conflicts	16	44
Transference material	37	62

(after Murray, 1962)

belief that relationship comes before the effectiveness of verbal reinforcement.

Why do I think this is important? I think what is happening is that as a clinical relationship is developed, it creates a possibility for a real extinction situation, in which anxiety is aroused in the presence of

TABLE 2

THE ACTIVITY AND PASSIVITY OF THERAPIST
REMARKS IN RELATION TO PATIENT
CONTENT CATEGORIES

Patient Content Categories	Percentage of Active Remarks	
	Case A	Case B
Psychotic symptoms	33	39
Family conflicts	33	27
Transference material	42	100

(after Murray, 1962)

someone important for the individual, and there is then anxiety extinction of an important and realistic nature. For instance, suppose a patient is talking about the fact that he is annoyed with his father. He knows he is sitting in an office and his father is 500 miles away. But it is much more realistic for him to sit there and say that he is annoyed with the therapist for being two minutes late (and the feelings are much more intense) than for him to say he is annoyed with his father. Extinction in this realistic situation is more likely to have an effect on the person's anxiety level in similar situations in real life.

47

In addition, I think the anxiety of the therapist is very important, can be communicated, and can slow down extinction. One of the reasons Rosen is fairly successful with schizophrenic patients, I believe, is that he does not seem to be afraid of them. Many people who work with schizophrenic patients go through a long period of having to overcome their own anxiety. There is also evidence suggesting special personality characteristics are associated with success with schizophrenics as opposed to neurotics. Other studies by Bandura (1956) suggest that approach-avoidance behavior on the part of patients is also related to the therapist's anxiety. He found that student therapists who had problems in the expression of hostility tended not to permit their patients to express hostility, particularly toward them. Since the patients' hostile feelings never came out, anxiety could not be extinguished. I see traditional therapy as being very much related to the arousal of anxiety concerning various things that have been bothering the patient, and a reduction in the anxiety through extinction.

NEWER FORMS OF PSYCHOTHERAPY

I should like to say a few things about other kinds of therapy and about theory not tied to the more traditional sort of therapy. Learning principles should be able to explain any kind of therapy from existential analysis to conditioning therapy. If behavior change is going on—if new learning is going on—then it should be accountable in these terms. Miller (1964) makes specific mention of other kinds of therapy and how they might be related to learning principles. One that he mentioned was Mowrer's superego therapy. Mowrer feels most of the emotional problems people face occur not because they are inhibited, but because they have transgressed and sinned. It is a deficit problem and they really have to inhibit certain kinds of behavior. Instead of there being too harsh a superego in Freudian terms, the superego may be too lenient.

Miller makes a distinction between realistic and unrealistic fears. He feels that if an individual is engaging in behavior in which there is a realistic fear of social retribution, the resolution lies in increasing, rather than reducing, the avoidance. The therapy I have described as traditional psychotherapy consists of reducing the avoidance component, for example, in the conflict model, through extinction. The avoidance is supposedly motivated by unrealistic fear or anxiety. If, in fact, one cannot get rid of punishment—if, in fact, society is very punitive—then

48

another option is to increase the avoidance so much the person is pushed entirely out of the conflict. Miller suggests this as another way of reducing conflict, and a person probably does suffer less when he is not torn in conflict.

My own feeling is that a lot of behavior that appears antisocial is really neurotic and motivated by feelings of inadequacy and fears of various kinds. For example, suppose a man masturbates a great deal and becomes guilt-ridden about this. It is possible that he engages in this behavior because he has a deeper conflict, a problem in relating to women. It would seem to me that one must concentrate on the more primary area and view the masturbation as a secondary phenomenon. So, too, many therapists go into great detail about a patient's homosexual behavior. Others, instead of concentrating on the fact that the patient is attracted to men, focus their attention on the fact that he cannot go out with women or that he cannot get married. The blocking of the heterosexual relationship is the important thing, because this may be the reason the patient turns in the homosexual direction. A number of therapists report that they get considerable success through concentrating on resolving the conflict in the heterosexual area.

Miller also suggests that radically different kinds of therapy can be explained by learning theory; for example, Albert Ellis' rational emotive therapy. I had the opportunity of hearing a tape from a case seen by Ellis. On the particular tape that I heard, a man came in and said he gets very depressed and was thinking of killing himself. Ellis said, as I remember, "Give me an example of when you feel this way," and the man replied something like, "Well, the other day the boss came in and he looked at my work and he said it was terrible. I went home and I felt depressed and I felt like shooting myself." Ellis replied, as I recall, "That is your trouble. Your trouble isn't that you get depressed; that is understandable. There is a missing link, there is a verbal formula that you have in between these two events. The verbal formula is that 'It is a catastrophe, it is terrible that he doesn't like my work!' As long as that little slogan or little verbal formula is in there, you are going to feel depressed, but it is not a catastrophe. Can you imagine my feeling upset if someone came in and said my work is no good? Can you imagine it bothering me?" Ellis has worked out about forty of these verbal formulae, such as, "Everybody has to love me" or "I have to be perfect" or "All of my work has to be perfect." In therapy he works with these mediating verbal responses. I think it is very important in a learning approach to try and understand the way in which verbal responses, the mediating verbal formulae that people use, control their emotions. Perhaps we can find ways, maybe better ways than Ellis', of breaking up these mediating responses, eliminating them. If we eliminate them we may eliminate the emotional reaction.

Then there is Wolpe's counterconditioning therapy.[2] Dr. Sanford Dean in our clinic at Syracuse University is very interested in this. A student therapist has used this procedure in working with a girl who had a snake phobia. First, the patient was seated in a very comfortable chair and instructed to relax. The topic of snakes was approached gradually. Initially, they only talked about animals in general. Then they talked about reptiles. Eventually, they talked about snakes as they looked at pictures. Finally, they went on a field trip to a zoology museum where they looked at stuffed snakes. There was to be a final step of having the patient actually touch a snake, but this was not done here. Nevertheless, I was impressed by the extent to which the subject's fears of snakes were diminished.

Another approach used by the behavior therapists is aversive conditioning. This is perhaps one of the oldest forms of learning therapy. For example, a procedure has been used with enuretics in which a bell rings if the bed becomes wet. This aversive conditioning has been used in England for rather delimited symptoms, and this may be of particular significance in the sense that stuttering is a fairly delimited symptom. I should like to mention one study on eliminating writer's cramps which points out the type of problem which can be involved in using aversive conditioning. Apparently, writer's cramps occurs in people who are very tense and who grasp the pencil very hard and press with tremendous pressure. One investigator (Beech, 1960) tried a procedure that involved having a pencil with a special arm that was wired so that the patient got an electric shock every time he pressed more than a certain amount. The main finding here was that with some groups of patients this was quite successful, but with others it was totally unsuccessful—as a matter of fact, the symptom worsened. With non-anxious individuals the electric shock helped eliminate the symptom, but people who were anxious got worse when they were shocked. I have some reservations about avoidance-conditioning procedures, because I think it depends to a very large extent on whether or not anxiety is involved. If a person is too anxious, certain of the procedures may be antitherapeutic.

2. Editor's note: For a description of this method of psychotherapy based on principles of learning, see Wolpe (1958).

CONCLUDING REMARKS

Psychotherapy may be viewed as a process of relearning. I have emphasized the importance of conflict reduction and anxiety extinction in traditional psychotherapy. I have also emphasized the *social* nature of the problems facing the psychotherapy patient and the *social* nature of the therapeutic relationship. Newer forms of psychotherapy are emerging and may hold great promise for the future, particularly if they come to terms with the problems of the patient in social living.

III

DEAN E. WILLIAMS

Stuttering Therapy: An Overview

THE SCIENTIFIC INVESTIGATION of the stuttering problem began approximately forty years ago. At that time stuttering, so to speak, was taken into the research laboratory.

Although it is always precarious to list "firsts," one can, with a fair degree of accuracy, state that the first systematic research programs were undertaken in the 1920's by Lee Travis and his students at the University of Iowa and by Robert West and his students at the University of Wisconsin. Much of the research done since that time has had as its primary purpose location of the cause of stuttering within the body or within the personality of the person who stuttered. Other studies have been done with the purpose of describing the conditions under which stuttering frequency increased or decreased. Still others were concerned with the interaction between the stutterer and persons in his environment.

52

Parallel with the continuous research programs have been numerous so-called theories about the cause and perpetuation of stuttering behavior. Some of the theories relied a great deal on research information for their bases and others for the most part ignored it. Persons with research interests in many different disciplines have contributed to the knowledge about the problem. Still others, with enthusiasm to match that of the researcher but not the scientific rigor, have hopped and skipped, often with free abandon, from technique to technique in an effort to solve the problem clinically. Neither discipline nor enthusiasm, methodical investigation nor imaginative theory has yet produced agreement among persons with different training and background as to the cause and perpetuation of stuttering. At this date, however, the most reliable information available points to the conclusion that stuttering is learned.

The cry for new ideas in the area of stuttering is becoming more intense. There is a perpetual search for a "new theory"—a new approach to the problem! At the same time, there is confusion as to the theories and approaches we now have and, too often, a lack of rigor in obtaining—or requiring—scientific data to support them. These comments are not to be construed as meaning that I am opposed to new ideas or to new theories. There is a need, however, to assess carefully, in systematic ways, and as completely as possible the information we have before we set out on our safari after "new" ideas. In fact, carefully assessing current information, asking new questions, and pondering relationships between known variables are the best routes to the development of new ideas.

I wish clinicians would place more stress on the asking of meaningful questions that can be answered by systematic observation. There is a tendency for too many clinicians to hurriedly sieve through convenient information in order to arrive at "answers." It is appalling to note the frequency with which such persons are seeking *only* "the answer." They scan new articles to see if they contain "the answer," they attend conferences and conventions with the hope of hearing "the answer." They spend relatively little time defining the questions to which they are attempting to seek answers. I am reminded of the time that I saw penciled on a wall the statement, "Faith is the answer." Scrawled underneath it was the notation, "Yes, I know, but what's the question?"

Operating in a spirit of "faith," some clinicians do not avail themselves of all pertinent information but instead wait for revelation. They look toward the so-called expert to provide answers for them to questions that they have never thought to ask. This kind of attitude produces an unhealthy effect in that it creates a temptation for the so-called expert, dazzled by his own "divinity," to reject the process of inquiry that we call scientific investigation. Such investigation could topple his throne of preconceived ideas, opinions, and clinical intuition.

The researcher and the clinician must work together. Neither is more important than the other. It will be through the systematic and careful observation that is a vital part of scientific method that the clinician will be able to define questions that can be and need to be answered. If the questions for which the researcher seeks answers are not meaningful, then the clinician is at fault for failing to provide the basis for meaningful questions. In order for the clinician to present meaningful questions he must become more systematic in the therapy that he does. He must become more interested in reporting in a scientific manner accounts of his principles and procedures of therapy. He must make clear statements of the basic assumptions about the nature of stuttering upon which he is operating. He must translate the available information into a systematic clinical program. Finally, he must methodically record clinical observations of the procedures he chooses. When the clinician has done these things, different principles and procedures of therapy can be compared, and we shall be in a position to formulate more meaningful questions. As more researchers begin answering the questions posed, the clinician's beliefs about the nature of the problem (beliefs around which his therapy program has been organized) will be based more and more on fact and less and less on faith.

It is recognized that the task of keeping systematic records of the principles and procedures used in therapy, and reporting these along with clinical observations of the client's behavior, will not be easy. Still it is obvious that a report of success—or lack of success—with a client is meaningless unless it occurs in conjunction with a description, insofar as possible, of the procedures used to obtain it.

THEORETICIAN AND CLINICIAN

While the researcher and theorist are concerned with the relationship of learning theories to stuttering behavior and formulate studies to test hypotheses, the clinician is immediately and directly concerned with learning and with learned behavior—figuratively speaking, "up to his neck," and little above. He is attempting to modify past learning and to institute new learning. His major questions revolve around the problem of the best ways to do this. In fact, the clinician can do little more in the clinical situation than help the stutterer change the things he has learned to do when he talks, the ways he has learned to feel and think about stuttering, and the ways he has learned to react to other people because of it.

The learning theorist and the clinician function using different criteria; they have different responsibilities, and they speak a different language. Bachrach, in the editor's introduction to *Experimental Foundations of Clinical Psychology,* points up these distinctions clearly. He quotes Dews (Bachrach, 1962), who states,

[clinical psychologists] are obligated constantly to make decisions as to the dispositions of their patients—decisions that usually cannot be solely or even primarily on the basis of available scientific evidence. It is the clear duty of the clinician to make this decision on the basis of all available information. It is the equally clear duty of the basic scientist *not* to come to a decision until scientific evidence justifies it. (p. 424)

Bachrach concludes:

The fundamental difference, then, lies in social obligations. Because a clinician must, out of human necessity, make decisions based on insufficient data, he is allowed a certain diplomatic immunity in his role on the ward. He is allowed such terms as "improvement," "therapy," "anxiety," without being required to specify the operational variables that go into them. The research psychologist, on the other hand, must assume the responsibilities, procedures, and criteria of the basic scientist. (p. ix)

Whereas it is obvious that to the learning theorist such terms as "avoidance conditioning" or "escape conditioning" or "operant conditioning" can be defined and hence have meaning only with regard to operational procedures, no such restrictions are placed on the clinician in this area. A considerable number of such "learning terms" have crept into the "language of stuttering." The clinician talks about avoidance, escape, conflict, and anxiety—just to mention a few. In clinical uses these terms have a variety of meanings depending upon the context in which they are used and the person who is using them. For example, to the research psychologist avoidance conditioning is a training procedure with specified variables in which the resultant learned reaction prevents the occurrence of a noxious stimulus. The clinician uses the term "avoidance behavior" in a descriptive sense to talk about the stuttering problem. The clinician may report that (1) a person who stutters often "avoids" the use of a word or a situation, (2) a person attempts to "avoid" stuttering as he talks, or (3) an instance of stuttering essentially is an "avoidance" reaction. Here, then, are three different meanings of the word "avoidance," none of which is directly comparable to the meaning ascribed to it by the research psychologist. One must exercise due caution in his use of the language of stuttering or he is likely to be lulled into thinking that clinicians are much more "learning theory oriented" than they really are.

Because of the fundamental differences between clinicians and theoreticians, it would be futile to attempt a systematic evaluation of the therapy procedures used in this country as they relate to learning theory. Furthermore, very little therapy research has been done and the data for comparisons are lacking.

Currently, investigation is under way into the possible use of operant conditioning procedures in stuttering or of Wolpe's desensitization type of behavior therapy. So far, results reported have been insufficient to permit meaningful evaluation. Preliminary reports, however, indicate that such procedures offer promise of being useful. Most certainly this kind of research is needed because, regardless of the results obtained, one will be able to describe the essential procedures used to obtain them.

THE CLINICIAN'S BELIEFS

Even though commonly used therapy procedures cannot be evaluated from a strict learning theory standpoint, they can be discussed from the standpoint of the ways in which the clinician's basic belief about the nature of the problem—his "theory" about the stuttering—affects the learning that takes place on the part of the client. It was stated previously that the clinician attempts to change behavior and attitudes that have been learned. In fact, that is all he can change. The principles and procedures commonly used to accomplish this have varied along a continuum. At one extreme is the clinician who is so hypnotized by the "surface noises" he hears that they are all he attempts to change. He apparently makes the assumption that if he changes these, the individual automatically will be able to change in other ways. The clinician at the opposite end of the continuum deals exclusively with the feelings and attitudes of the stutterers. He usually does this in a counseling-type therapy situation. Apparently he makes the assumption that if these feelings and attitudes are changed, corresponding changes in speaking behavior automatically will follow. The majority of clinicians today, however, fall at various points between these two extremes. Where the

56

clinician falls on this continuum depends upon his basic beliefs about the nature of the stuttering problem.

One hears with increasing regularity the statement that clinicians differ in their opinions about the cause of stuttering, but when they begin doing therapy, they do substantially the same thing. If this is correct, then I should stop my paper at this point and merely make the statement that most clinicians are in substantial agreement and hence do essentially the same thing in therapy. It is my belief, however, that this assumption is based on a misconception. Two clinicians may use the same technique but give different instructions and information to the client. The two clients therefore will *learn* different things by applying the dissimilar instructions and information received. What each *learns* is the essence of therapy—the technique is not.

For example, a stutterer may be asked to talk to a clerk in a store and to practice remaining calm while stuttering openly. This may be done for a variety of reasons: He may be asked to observe (1) his internal feelings of hostility toward the clerk, (2) that he feels better when he does not "avoid" stuttering, (3) that his "spasms" are not as frequent or severe when he remains relatively calm, (4) that his "block" is easier to control when he remains calm, (5) that it is easier for him to evaluate the behavior he is using to interfere with talking if he remains relatively calm, and the like. The things he will learn will depend upon the ways the problem has been explained to him and the kinds of specific questions he is attempting to answer or the observations he is supposed to make. These questions or observations will vary considerably depending upon a clinician's assumptions about the variables affecting the problem.

It works something like this: Before a clinician can begin to do stuttering therapy meaningfully, he must assess his own beliefs about the nature of stuttering. Once he does this, he formulates a retraining program that *is related* to the basic concepts that he holds about the nature of the problem. He adopts a language in talking about the problem. He devises procedures that he believes will achieve his goals of therapy.

This question of "What do I believe constitutes the problem of stuttering?" is forced into sharp focus when the clinician faces across the clinical desk a person who stutters and who has come to him for help. The clinician begins to structure the clinical situation so the client can start to change his attitudes, beliefs, and behavior. How does the clinician begin? First of all he makes observations about the ways the individual is talking, the ways he is interacting with people in his environment, and the ways he feels about himself and about other people. The process of sorting out the individual's behavior and then assessing the significance of it depends to a great extent on the ways the clinician understands the nature of the problem. One cannot divorce the two.

It is possible to describe the stutterer's behavior with a minimum of interpretation as to its underlying meaning and to group the descriptions in a variety of ways. One category of such descriptions might be based on what the clinician sees the stutterer do as he talks. This can result in a listing of such things as articulatory postures, straining facial movements, muscle tensings, and the like. Another set of listings might be based on descriptions of what the clinician hears the stutterer do as he talks. These include such things as repeating sounds, prolonging a sound, rising inflection, and prolonged periods of silence. A third category would be to describe the stutterer's general bodily behavior as he interacts with people. This could include a description of the tensing of arms and legs, of fidgeting in a chair, or of excessive perspiration. Still another set of listings is to describe the language that a stutterer uses to talk about himself and the world around him. This could include the language he uses in talking about his own behavior, in talking about the ways he gets along with other people, and in talking about the ways he views himself in relation to other people—his fears and beliefs about his relationships with people. A final category could be a listing of the ways the stutterer feels, of embarrassments, shame, and guilt about the ways he talks.

In fact, though, most clinicians do not merely collect behavioral data. As they obtain information about how the stutterer behaves, most clinicians begin to assess the *significance* or the *meaning* of what they see or of what they hear. The clinician ascribes meaning *to* this behavior and then begins to develop a retraining program in conjunction with the interpretation that he makes about the importance of what he has seen and what he has heard the individual do. The meanings the clinician ascribes to the behavior—that is, the interpretations that he makes—depend upon the basic assumptions that he has about the nature of the problem or, to say it simply, his theory about stuttering. Clinicians observe the individual behaving through the filters of their own beliefs.

For example, the clinician may describe the stutterer's speech as being characterized by repetitions and some facial tensing. This is purely a *description* of the way the individual was behaving. Then, however, the clinician may go on and say that these repetitions and facial tensings are serving to postpone or to avoid or to conceal some other kind of behavior. These statements are *evaluations* by the clinician of the significance of the behavior described. If the clinician is operating within a theory involving "avoidance and postponement," he is likely to say that the person is tensing in an effort to avoid or postpone the saying of the word because of the fear of stuttering, or of repeating. If his orientation is more "psychological," he may say that the individual is repeating and tensing in order to cover up hostility. If, on the other hand, the clinician's orientation is one in which he believes there is a neurological deficit, he is likely to say that the repeating is part of the "primary stutter" and that the tensings are merely "secondary reactions" to it. It would be possible to continue with many other kinds of interpretations, but I believe that my point is clear: the explanation that the clinician transmits to the client affects the kinds of things the client learns as he becomes further involved in therapy.

There is certainly sufficient evidence of verbal conditioning to indicate that a person's behavior can be influenced by subtle kinds of reinforcement. The clinician's eyes may light up or he may lean forward in his chair, or he may respond with "m-hmm" when the client begins mentioning some aspect of his behavior that the clinician feels is important in relation to the problem. If the clinician responded in such fashion when the client mentioned the fact that he was unhappy about some aspect of his mother's behavior toward him, it is entirely likely that the client would dwell more and more on aspects of his mother's behavior. Then the clinician would arrive at the conclusion, "I was right, his mother's behavior was important—he can talk about little else."

The *meaning* given to an individual's behavior is based on the clinician's interpretation and is not inherent within the individual's behavior. These comments are not meant to be a criticism of the clinician who reacts in these ways (inasmuch as we are human, we all tend to act this way). The point is made in an attempt to show that a clinician, no matter how vaguely defined his assumptions may be, *does* have a theory about the nature of the problem. He must recognize what that theory is and what effect it has in his therapy.

Only when the clinician knows what his theory is can he maintain a consistent direction in therapy. If he does not have an explicit hypothesis, it is easy for him to read any book or any article that may appear in print and abstract a technique here and a technique there to use in therapy without any realization that there is a need to integrate and unite

59

them. If a clinician is confused about his hypothesis, or if he has never stopped to evaluate what it might be, it is predictable that he will be inconsistent and confused in therapy. Too often the clinician is concerned with *what* to do in therapy instead of *why* one wants to do it. Such preoccupation with method can result in an incongruity between what the clinician considers to be the nature of the problem and what he does in therapy. The result is extreme difficulty in evaluating the effectiveness of the therapy program. Only when procedures are chosen in the light of beliefs can the clinician evaluate the effectiveness of his therapy program and, if necessary, re-evaluate his basic assumptions about the problem.

If it is the clinician's goal to make the stutterer "feel better" about his problem and to "adjust to it," then he should recognize this and use every technique he can to achieve that goal. If the results are not too effective, he should re-examine his basic concept about the problem and not proceed by merely adopting new procedures of therapy indiscriminately simply because they might help. If it is the clinician's basic belief that there is something "organically wrong" with the stutterer, that he always will be a stutterer, and that, consequently, he should work to control as best he can his stuttering behavior and try for an objective attitude about it, then the clinician should develop procedures that can best accomplish this goal. If his results are not satisfying, then he, too, should re-examine his basic assumptions about the nature of the problem and the language he uses in talking about it. He should not simply adopt some new clinical procedures irrespective of the assumptions out of which they are born and intermingle them with some of his old ones simply because of a hope born out of desperation that they might work. Being sure that his procedures derive logically from his hypotheses is the most meaningful way that a clinician has, at the present time, of employing the scientific method in evaluating his assumptions and procedures.

Some people will question the feasibility of the clinician's employing scientific methods. This doubt is due to the usual meaning given to the word "science." It is thought of too often as a body of knowledge, or an elaborately equipped laboratory, or a man in a white coat. "Scientific method" is used in this paper as Wendell Johnson referred to it in *People in Quandaries* (1946). He states:

. . . the method of science consists in (a) asking clear, answerable questions in order to direct one's (b) observations, which are made in a calm and unprejudiced manner, and which are then (c) reported as accurately as possible in such a way as to answer the questions that were asked to begin with, after which (d) any pertinent beliefs or assumptions that were held before the observations were made are revised in light of the observations made and the answers obtained. Then more questions are asked in accordance with the newly revised notions, further observations are made, new answers are arrived at, beliefs and assumptions are again revised, after which the whole process starts over again. In fact, it never stops. Scientific method is continuous. All its conclusions are held subject to further revision that new observations may require. It is the method of keeping one's information, beliefs, and theories up to date. It is, above all, a method of "changing one's mind"—sufficiently often. (p. 49)

INTEGRATION OF THEORY AND THERAPY

The need to integrate scientific method into a clinical approach toward stuttering is well illustrated in a most interesting chapter by Charles Van Riper entitled "A Brief History of the Treatment of Stuttering." It appears in the book, *Stuttering: Research and Therapy,* edited by Joseph Sheehan (1968). Van Riper summarizes some of the theories and therapies of stuttering reported between the 1700's and the present time. From the point of view of philosophy toward therapy, the years he covered in his review of the literature can be divided into two periods: from the 1700's to 1925 and from 1925 to the present. The 1925 date corresponds roughly with the beginning of the work of Lee Travis and Robert West mentioned earlier.[1] Up to 1925 the philosophy toward therapy can be best expressed as an antistuttering approach. The philosophy of therapy after 1925 can be thought of as the antianxiety approach.

In the antistuttering approach of the pre-1925 period, the main purpose was to encourage the stutterer to apply some technique to "keep from stuttering." Phonetic drills, rate control, rhythmic timing procedures, and the like were used. These techniques remained in use throughout the period despite the fact that the thinking about the causes of stuttering changed greatly. It is interesting to note the frequency with which an individual would propose a new theory about the cause of stuttering but then would employ the same techniques in therapy that had been used for years before that time. In other words, it often appears that a therapeutic technique, once introduced, gallops along through history independent of, and often completely unrelated to, theory about the cause of the stuttering.

The antianxiety approach adopted after 1925 aimed, not at eliminating stuttering, but at reducing the struggling behavior and the anxiety

61

about it. Acceptance of this approach to stuttering therapy coincides roughly with the introduction of the cerebral dominance theory by Travis and Orton and the dysphemia theory by West, which had in common the assumption that there was an organic cause for stuttering. From this assumption—namely, that an organic cause existed—it logically followed that the best therapy procedure would be one which would help the person to accept the fact that he stuttered and to help him become less anxious about it and "do a good easy job of stuttering." It is important to note that the therapy procedures introduced at that time are still very much with us today. Clinicians are still operating within this same philosophy even though there have been many changes in theoretical positions.

My purpose is not to evaluate the appropriateness or inappropriateness of any technique. It is to alert the clinician to the need to weigh the therapy procedures he uses and to question the reasons that he uses them. Do they correspond to his basic beliefs about stuttering, or are they merely techniques used because "that is the way one works with stuttering"? My point can be illustrated by examining a little more closely, as an example, the cerebral dominance theory and citing some of the concepts out of which therapy procedures developed. The clinician using these therapy procedures at the present time should evaluate them as to whether the reasons for which they were introduced are the reasons that they are in use now. If so, fine. If not, what is the rationale for using them? If there is one, fine. If not, why not?

In essence, the cerebral dominance theory held that the stutterer possessed a different type of neuro-organization than did a normal person. It was thought that he lacked a dominant controlling and integrating mechanism in the cerebral cortex sufficient to withstand the disintegrating effect of emotional stress. Among those factors supposed to contribute to the lack of dominance was a shift in handedness, ordinarily forced upon the child at a fairly early age. As a result, there was emphasis on shifting the handedness of the individual back under the control of the presumably dominant hemisphere and efforts were made to help the person to increase the threshold of breakdown under emotional stress. If, as it was hypothesized, the speaking mechanism broke down under stressful social situations, then it was logical to help the stutterer withstand such stress. In addition, it was held that the stuttering act itself produced an emotionally stressful situation that resulted in additional breakdown in speech behavior.

On the basis of this theory, therapy was seen as having two major goals. One goal was to help the person understand that he was a stutterer, that there was nothing he could do about it in a basic sense, and that, therefore, he must learn to accept it. This resulted in considerable emphasis on the so-called objective attitude by which the person could learn to accept himself as a stutterer. The second major goal was to help the person stutter as easily and as effortlessly and as unobtrusively as possible. This was done for two reasons: (1) so his listeners would not react unduly to his stuttering and by their reaction cause additional anxiety and stress; and (2) so he would not feel as badly about it, and hence it would not trigger additional stuttering. Therefore, the person would work to modify and to simplify his stuttering, to accept it, and to learn to stutter or "have his spasm" in an easy and effortless way. In brief, the goals were to reduce anxiety, to reduce emotional reaction, and to reduce the complexity and the severity of the "stutterer."

Today many students of the problem assume that stuttering is learned behavior. Helping the individual accept "the fact" that he is a stutterer and always will be one and striving to decrease the "stutter" so he can stutter easily are not consistent with the ways we tend to work with other kinds of learned behavior.

In certain respects, therefore, it would appear that even though clinicians have ceased shifting handedness and seldom use the word "dysphemia" anymore, they have maintained the basic principles of therapy that were derived from an organic theory.

Confusion has also been produced by the language we use to talk about stuttering. Much of this language was introduced as a way of talking about the problem in conjunction with a neurological cause. For example, one may hear a clinician discuss the "secondary reactions" of a particular stutterer. The term "secondary reactions" was used frequently in conjunction with the neurological explanation because it implied that a primary or basic "stutter" was there inside the individual and would occur regardless of what the stutterer did. It "happened" particularly if he was in a stressful situation. It was hypothesized that in this type of situation, the individual would react by struggling to cover up, to conceal, or to "hold to a minimum" the basic or primary stuttering. This, of course, implies a neurological or in some fashion an organic cause, with the struggling merely secondary reactions to it. In this context there are important distinctions between the theoretical positions of different persons. From the neurological viewpoint there is a "stutter" separate from the speaker's strugglings and reactions to it. It is these secondary

63

reactions—the strugglings—that have been learned. Another position is that the behavior we label stuttering is made up entirely of a learned reaction pattern. Without taking sides at this point, I am bound to say it does not appear logical that one would proceed in therapy in the same ways regardless of which position was held. The fact that clinicians of the two schools of thought may follow similar procedures should cause us to pause and examine some of our basic beliefs about the problem and then to examine the consistency and the logic of the retraining procedures that we use.

If, for a moment, another kind of behavior is considered, perhaps the point about the language we use will be clarified. Most clinicians at one time or another have worked with an individual who produces a lateral /s/. There is no implication intended by the use of this example that I consider the problem of a lateral /s/ and stuttering to be directly comparable. I wish to use this example, however, to point out a general orientation that clinicians assume when they consider behavior to be learned and that they do not assume when they do not consider it to be learned. The example of the lateral /s/ is used simply because most people basically believe that this is learned. In lateral /s/ therapy, then, the general orientation is toward learning. Clinicians most certainly would not work with a person to any great extent to have him accept himself as a "lateral /s/er." They would not consider the lateral /s/ to be a secondary reaction to a primary lateral /s/. Moreover, they would not work on the behavior by helping him to decrease his lateral /s/ or to simplify his lateral /s/. There would be no attempt to help him learn to "control" his lateral /s/. Instead, clinicians are much more positive. They help him become aware of the procedures for making a good /s/ sound and then they help him work in that direction. They reinforce the good /s/ sound. They do not reinforce a "less bad" /s/ sound. In fact, it would never occur to clinicians to talk about it that way.

My point here is one of philosophy, an attitude toward attempting to change behavior. The general philosophy during the past forty years has required that the clinician in the stuttering area be a "decreaser" or a "controller" of certain kinds of undesirable behavior. Yet, when a clinician is faced with other behavior that is readily accepted as being learned, he takes the position of being an "increaser of desirable behavior."

One must be aware of the language he uses in talking about the stuttering problem because language is a powerful vehicle for perpetuating a frame of reference, a way of thinking, without one's ever being

64

aware that his language is doing his thinking for him. The language used in discussing stuttering actually *promotes* a belief that stuttering is one thing and the individual struggling and tensing behavior is something else—a reaction to the "stuttering." Within this frame of reference, the question of how do one's reactions differ from the "real" stuttering is a very perplexing one. This perplexity is due as much to the language as it is to any "unexplainable mystery" about the problem of stuttering.

CLIENT'S BELIEFS AND EXPECTATIONS

Up to this point I have emphasized the effect that philosophy has on the clinician. It is important also to consider in more detail the effect that it has on the client. The ways in which the client learns to talk to himself are going to define, in part, the kinds of changes he believes he can make. Farber (1963) made an especially important comment in this regard in his discussion of the role of "awareness" in verbal conditioning. He stated:

Subjects may not know exactly what is going on in an experiment or, for that matter, in therapeutic sessions, but very few have no ideas at all. They may be mistaken, or they may be concerned with irrelevant matters, such as whether participation in the experiment is worth the time and trouble, or whether the counselor is as blasé as he seems, or what is for lunch. The one thing psychologists can count on is that their subjects or clients will talk, if only to themselves. And, not infrequently, whether relevant or irrelevant, the things people say to themselves determine the rest of the things they do.

There is little doubt that what the stutterer does and what he comes to expect to be able to do are determined in part by the way he talks to himself. It is in this way that he comes to define his problem to himself and subsequently acts upon it.

For example, a stutterer is likely to learn in therapy, by means of mirror work and self-analysis, that he holds his breath *when he stutters,* he tenses his jaw *when he stutters,* and he blinks his eyes *when he stutters.* This kind of language implies that these behaviors accompany the stuttering. In other words he does them when a "stuttering" occurs. Then, it is within this context that the stutterer is asked to "control" these "secondary reactions" to the stutter. It is interesting to speculate upon whether or not—if the stutterer could eliminate the holding of breath, the tensing of jaw, the blinking of eyes, the repeating of sounds, and so forth—the "stutter" would still remain. If it remained what would it be? How would it be discernible? A language that is more consistent

65

with the concept that stuttering is learned would be one in which the client learns that he holds his breath *as he talks,* he tenses his jaw *as he talks,* he blinks his eyes *as he talks,* and so forth. Implied in this kind of language is that if he changes these behaviors, all that is left is talking.

CONCLUSION

We as clinicians need to (a) evaluate our basic assumptions about the nature of the stuttering problem and weigh these assumptions against available information; (b) develop principles and procedures of therapy—and a language to talk about them—consistent with a basic assumption about the nature of the problem; (c) keep systematic records of therapy sessions so that the procedures followed and the results obtained can be evaluated in a logical way; and (d) pose pertinent questions for the researcher to answer.

IV

O. HOBART MOWRER

Stuttering as Simultaneous

Admission and Denial; *or,*

What Is the Stutterer "Saying"?

THE READER SHOULD BE FOREWARNED that this paper [1] is almost wholly speculative—or, perhaps more precisely, inferential and deductive. In other words, the point of view which will be set forth herein is but a special case or application of an overarching conception of psychopathology in general. The author (and his students) have, to be sure, had stutterers as patients; but this has been relatively rare—and the results, again relatively speaking, modest. However, the intractability of the symptom, as will be indicated later, may be a confirmation of the proposed explanation, rather than a negation of it.

1. Editor's note: Dr. Mowrer presented this material in the Symposium on Stuttering at Northwestern University in August, 1965. Subsequently, a paper based on this lecture was published in the *Journal of Communication Disorders* (Mowrer, 1967). Appreciation is expressed to the editor, Robert Rieber, for granting permission to reproduce this article in essentially the same form in which it appeared in the *Journal.*

Freud and the Freudians have long emphasized the "biphasic" nature of symptoms. Due to the excessive counterforce of moral scruple (i.e., the superego), some impulse (such as sex or aggression) is, they hold, "repressed," in the sense of being not only denied overt expression and gratification but also of being excluded from representation in consciousness. As long as the repression is maintained, the repudiated impulse will, of course, continue to clamor and strive for satisfaction, but satisfaction will be possible only if it is *disguised* and also accompanied by *suffering*. Thus, the Freudians have held that symptoms involve both an element of distorted ("displaced") instinctual pleasure *and* "moral" pain. But since the pain is fully explicit and the gratification much less so, the symptom is seen as primarily painful—and therefore mysterious.

If the symptom is as painful as the patient reports, why does it persist? Freud's conjecture was that the motivating force behind a symptom is always instinctual, in the way already indicated. The element of gratification, he maintained, is also always present; but it is more or less camouflaged to begin with and is then overlaid by suffering to make it more acceptable. The "symptom" thus persists because, in balance, it is rewarding.[2]

Perhaps it is thus legitimate to say that Freud "discovered the unconscious," but it is far less certain that he ever understood what is *in it*. Efforts to alleviate symptoms, prevent "neurosis," and provide sound guidance to the good life which have been predicated on Freudian assumptions have, by and large, borne bitter fruit; and at this juncture we have, it would seem, no choice but to search for more felicitous conceptions.

There is today mounting experimental as well as clinical evidence (Mowrer, 1961, 1964, 1965a, 1965b) for believing that in "neurosis" the instinctual pleasure which is causing the trouble is not a mere "dangerous" *wish* which might be gratified in the future but a grim reality, a *fact* of the past. It is quite astonishing how completely would-be therapists and other clinical investigators have, in our time, looked for subtle indications of repressed impulses and systematically ignored a long history of socially inappropriate *impulse satisfaction*. And the result of such a life style is *guilt*, which, as a good first approxima-

2. However, Freud resolved this horn of the dilemma only to find himself impaled upon the other one: if, as he maintained, the moral fears which impede normal, direct impulse expression are excessive and unrealistic, why do these fears not spontaneously extinguish? In other words, the question is: Why are not all "neuroses" self-correcting?

tion, can be defined as a chronic fear of being found out and punished (as would have happened if the individual had been "caught in the act").

Immediately, of course, an important distinction has to be made between individuals who, because of poor character, can experience only "sociological" or "objective" guilt (i.e., the fear of being caught and punished by others), *and* individuals who, because of basically good character, are subject to the judgment and harassment of that inner tribunal we call conscience. The first type of individual is, of course, the "sociopath"; and the second type is the "neurotic" or, more appropriately, the "psychopath" (if the word had not previously been used for the sociopath), because the trouble is now psychic, in the intrapersonal rather than interpersonal sense.

Thus, for the person of poor character, wrongdoing leads to conflict only if he is caught and confronted by others; whereas, in the person of good character, wrongdoing sets up an *inner* conflict, regardless of whether he is socially apprehended or not. In this type of person, society has, so to say, a "secret agent" or "representative in residence," and the "crime" does not have to be known on the outside for outside influences to start having an effect. (This, of course, is the reason we try to give all children a conscience: so they will have inner controls and, hopefully, not get into "trouble with the law," in the objective sense of the term.)

Ordinarily, when we behave in a way which is socially (morally) inappropriate but not yet externally known, conscience, as we say, "speaks to us" or "protests." Now the individual faces a critical decision: Will he do the behest of conscience—confess, make restitution, and amend his ways? Or will he ignore conscience and persevere in a policy of duplicity and "hardness of heart"? If the individual chooses the latter course of action (and here we are assuming that human beings do have choice in such matters—see Cherbonnier, 1955), what *then* is conscience to do? What, we may ask, would an "ambassador" in the international sphere do in such an instance? Manifestly he would try to get "word" back to the country he represents, in the hope of getting "outside" assistance. But now let us further suppose that the offending "foreign" country decides to close all "diplomatic channels" and not let the damaging report or criticism "get out."

The personal condition we ambiguously call "neurosis" is, I submit, analogous. Conscience begins to try to get the "report" out, but the individual (in Sullivan's sense of "ego system") resolves to suppress it. For a time, there may be a sort of stalemate, reflected only by lowered personal efficiency, since the individual must now spend so much time guarding against a "slip" or "leak" of some sort. But eventually, if conscience is reasonably strong and persevering, it manages to interfere with or distort ongoing action in such a way as to make the individual's behavior very strange and suspicious. Anyone can then see that something is manifestly "wrong" with the afflicted person, but he continues to try to keep the exact nature of his "problem" from being known. This "compromise formation"—between a desire (on the part of conscience) for communication *and* a desire (on the part of the ego) for concealment—is, I believe, the essential dynamism of all neurotic symptoms.

Now we must ask: Is stuttering a "symptom"? Because of its common intractability to conventional therapeutic approaches, many writers have maintained that it is not; and I am not here prepared to argue very forcibly otherwise. All I ask is that we be willing to *consider* it in the light of the conception of neurosis which has just been sketched. And if we do this, we see that stuttering (as well as other "functional speech disorders") has a special status among symptoms: it is an especially *good* one, in that conscience has succeeded in getting its message into the individual's main communication channel in such a way that, if the message itself cannot be clearly transmitted, it can at least "jam" and distort what the ego or self-system is trying to say. That is, although the ego stubbornly refuses to let conscience tell its story directly, conscience can, if strong and clever enough, seriously interfere with what the ego is trying to "tell the world"—and thus provide a broad hint that something on the "inside" is not as it should be.

When conscience is able to produce only "bodily" symptoms, its message is inchoate and only remotely intelligible. But when it manages to get into the nervous centers controlling speech, this is extraordinarily good from the standpoint of conscience—and very bad, very dangerous as far as the self-system is concerned.

At the outset of this paper, I said that stuttering has proved intractable to therapeutic efforts which have been predicated on this kind of thinking. I now realize that "intractable" is not quite the correct term. What I should say instead is that, without exception so far as I can recall, stutterers who have sought this type of therapy (without perhaps understanding what they were getting into) have not continued. Several instances immediately come to mind in which the patient simply disappeared as soon as the therapist began to "hear" what his speech impediment was "saying." For example, I recall a Jewish college boy from a devout family who said, quite frankly, that he would rather stutter a little (his incapacity was indeed relatively slight) than to tell his parents (a) that he had long made a practice of pilfering small amounts of money from his father's wallet, and (b) that he now occasionally joins his fraternity brothers in visits to a house of prostitution in a nearby town. The embarrassment of not being able to *talk properly* was, apparently, sufficient atonement to prevent this young man from becoming seriously "decompensated." And we may also conjecture that conscience in this instance felt (if one may speak in such a vein) that, in producing such an "obvious" symptom as stuttering, it had already done its duty and that it was now up to others to "get the message" and decide what should be done about the situation.

My surmise is that if a stutterer could be *kept* in "therapy" of this kind, he could be "cured." If this is not true, either the whole conception of psychotherapy which has here been delineated is invalid, *or* stuttering is not, after all, a "neurotic symptom." Flanagan, Goldiamond, and Azrin (1959) have suggested that stuttering is a "habit" which, like any other habit, has come into existence, not because of any such complicated reasons as suggested here, but because of a history of systematic positive reinforcement. And in support of this thesis these investigators report that verbal nonfluency can be reliably increased in otherwise normal speakers by standard behavior-shaping (Skinnerian) methods.

What are the implications of this finding for the hypothesis suggested in the foregoing pages? The hypothesis set forth in this paper, it should be said, is not without adumbrations in the clinical literature on stuttering. Wischner (1950) and Sheehan (1953a) have both published related suggestions; and I am sure that anyone who is more conversant with the "speech" literature than I am could find other instances of related theorizing. The present paper, as indicated at the outset, is very schematic and claims empirical support only indirectly; in other words, as a special case of a general conception of psychopathology which seems to be steadily gaining in credibility.

V

JOSEPH SHEEHAN

Stuttering as a Self-Role Conflict

A CONFLICT OF STATUS AND ROLE

STUTTERING IS A FALSE-ROLE DISORDER. It is not a speech problem per se, but an interpersonal communication disorder. It is a fault in the social presentation of the self, a self-role conflict. As a species of approach-avoidance conflict, stuttering revolves around two chief factors: the self variable and the role variable.

First let us consider the self variable: The occurrence of stuttering is a function of how the individual feels toward himself in general, and how he feels particularly in his role as a speaker. For stuttering is *role-specific* behavior. Except in his role as speaker, the stutterer is not so different from other people. The concept of role specificity with reference to stuttering is immensely clarifying. The man who said that he stuttered only when he talked neatly illustrates the role-specific character of the problem. Behaviorally speaking, and in terms of any available measure,

72

the stutterer is a stutterer only when he talks. When he is not talking, when he is not stuttering, he is like anyone else. The feeling that the stutterer has about himself, especially in the speaker role, seems to be crucial to the occurrence of stuttering. This, then, is the first factor, the self variable.

The second factor, the role variable, refers to relationships, to status—in G. H. Mead's term, the "significant other" (Mead, 1934), the listener with whom communication is attempted. What is the stutterer's attitude toward that other person? What is the interpersonal relationship? This is the second great variable in stuttering.

So you stutter depending upon (1) how you feel toward yourself, upon the speaker variable; and (2) how you feel toward the other person, the listener variable. Stuttering is thus a conflict which is both intrapersonal and interpersonal. It is intrapersonal in that it revolves around one's own defenses, upon the self. It is interpersonal in that it is largely a disorder of social relations.

One of the most significant things we can say about a stutterer is that when he is alone he has little or no trouble. A few stutterers seem to project an audience for themselves, and report that they stutter to some extent even when alone. But such cases are rare, and it is uniformly reported by stutterers that they have little difficulty without a listener other than themselves. In other words, stuttering requires both a speaker and a listener.

The Status-Gap Hypothesis

The stutterer is most likely to block when he feels low in self-esteem, least likely to block when he feels high in self-esteem. He is most likely to stutter when he is in awe of the listener, or when the listener is a significant person, or when there is some conflict in the relationship, or when there is threat of penalty for stuttering.

Two studies, one involving the role variable and the other the self variable, may be cited as experimental support for the status-gap hypothesis and for the theory of stuttering as a self-role conflict.

To study the effect of authority "role demand," [1] thirty-two adult stutterers read matched passages to authority listeners and to peer listeners. Authority listeners were Ph.D. faculty members introduced by

1. For a general presentation of role theory concepts and related research, see (Sarbin, 1943, 1954).

title, and peer listeners were fellow college students introduced by first name (Sheehan, Hadley, and Gould, 1967).

The two chief findings of the study were that stutterers have more difficulty speaking to authority listeners, and that they have more trouble adapting to them over time. Both the initial frequency of stuttering and the rate of decline in frequency appear to be at least in part a function of the authority variable.

When combined with the finding of Bardrick and Sheehan (1956) on the effect on stuttering frequency of emotionally loaded material that poses a threat to the stutterer's self-esteem, these findings provide support for the "status-gap" hypothesis. Stuttering appears to vary as a function of the perceived status of the self, the speaker, and of the significant other, the listener. The lower the self-esteem of the speaker, or the more authority-laden the status of the listener, the more stuttering. A clear implication for therapy with stutterers is that among major goals would be change in the self-concept and change in relation to others— goals perhaps common to nearly all but the most mechanically oriented psychotherapies.

APPROACH-AVOIDANCE CONFLICT IN STUTTERING

Self and role conflicts are examples of conflict levels in stuttering. Conflict levels have been presented thoroughly as a part of previous publications of the approach-avoidance conflict theory of stuttering (Sheehan, 1953a, 1958b). The self variable was partially covered in connection with the ego-protective level of conflict, and the role variable was partially discussed in connection with relationship-level conflict.

Nothing in the foregoing sections, viewing stuttering in social psychological and role theory terms, should be construed as downgrading in any way the central importance of approach-avoidance conflict theory as explanatory of stuttering. The theoretical model is taken partly from Lewin (1936), but principally from Miller (1944), and from Dollard and Miller (1950). Further discussion of the model may be found in Murray's chapter in this volume.

Reduced to the simplest behavioral terms, stuttering is a momentary blocking. The stutterer halts, then gets started again. These are twin features of the stutterer's behavior for which any theory must account. For a while, the individual is stuck. Then he goes through the strange kind of behavior called "stuttering." The behavior itself is curiously unrelated to the phonetic production of the word. The stutterer may nod his head, snap his fingers, in saying, "My name is . . uh . . (nod) . . uh . . (snap) . . uh . . Joe." Why should he be any better able to say the word after he has gone through this little ritual? Why should saying "uh" or making sudden movements of head or hands seemingly permit the word to be said? This is perhaps an example of past operant conditioning, what Skinner (1948) has called superstitious behavior as applied to pigeons.

The stutterer has learned to do certain things that are self-distracting or disinhibiting. He gets a constant inflow of suggestions from people who say, "relax, and think what you have to say," "take a deep breath," "talk with marbles in your mouth," and he's tempted to try each new suggestion.

One of the important things to know about stuttering is that anything the stutterer tries will work for a while. Sheer novelty will seem for a time to help. This makes the investigation of stuttering enormously complex, and leads to endless anecdotes about the wonderful little gimmicks that supposedly cure stuttering.

Growing up as a severe stutterer, I would hear such stories almost daily, starting with the legend of Demosthenes' pebbles. After trying everything else, I did attempt to talk with pebbles myself once. I didn't quite believe the legend, but I felt I should leave no stones untried. I almost swallowed the pebbles and quickly resumed the search for new crutches.

Since any new distraction or fresh ritual temporarily suppresses stuttering, proponents abound for all varieties of bizarre therapy. Even the Delacato approach has been tried (Delacato, 1963). The stutterer, who has self-esteem problems anyway, is asked, of all things, to crawl because he stutters! For a worse approach than this we would have to go back more than one hundred years, to the surgical mutilation of the tongue.

Not only is stuttering susceptible to distraction, to suggestion, to little hypnotic influences, but the behavior is highly sensitive to all sorts of nuances in the social situation. Relative status of speaker and listener is but one of these.

Stuttering, Homeostasis, and Reinforcement

We must understand and explain how a set of behaviors so unattractive and obviously unadaptive as those we find in stuttering patterns manage to continue, apparently almost on a self-maintaining, self-reinforcing, or functionally autonomous basis. Why doesn't the behavior called stuttering extinguish? When it does not, what is the nature and source of reinforcement for these behaviors?

Stuttering is equally puzzling in terms of the principle of homeostasis. As developed by Cannon, homeostasis relates to the effort of the organism to maintain a kind of physiological equilibrium. We tend to react to physiological disturbance in such a way as to minimize it. On a psychological level, at least, the stutterer seems not to follow the principle of homeostasis. He reacts to his disturbance, e.g., his stuttering behavior, in such a way as to make it worse. He forces, or struggles, or strains, and makes speech production more difficult for himself. So here is a further puzzle in reconciling stuttering behavior with certain general principles of behavior.

Although the behavior of an individual stutterer may seem to be all mystery and hodgepodge, a series of randomly learned instrumental acts, actually there is systematization, lawfulness, and internal consistency in such behavior.

Stuttering is thus puzzling in terms of the twin principles of reinforcement and homeostasis. If it is behavior more punishing than rewarding, why is it continued? In earlier writings, Mowrer (1948) called this dilemma the neurotic paradox. Why should anybody persist in behavior that is apparently neurotic or non-reinforcing? In learning theory terms, what is the source of the reinforcement? What keeps the behavior going?

The Conflict Hypothesis and the Fear-Reduction Hypothesis

To be complete, any theory of stuttering must account first for the fact that the stutterer gets stuck. He gets blocked for some reason that is quite mysterious. Then, for a reason that is equally mysterious, he is able to go on. Why should this be?

Two hypotheses have been advanced to account for these twin features of stuttering behavior: (1) the conflict hypothesis; and (2) the fear-reduction hypothesis.

The Conflict Hypothesis. The stutterer blocks or stops because the forces for approaching the act of speaking and those for holding back from the act of speaking are temporarily in equilibrium. That is, he wants to speak, he has something to say, something to express, but he holds back. We all go through this kind of conflict. Anyone who has ever tried to explain his behavior when feeling guilty, or has tried to talk a traffic policeman out of a ticket, or has tried to explain himself when cast in an unfavorable role finds himself faltering in speech. Even the best of speakers will under such circumstances tend to have difficulty.

We all respond to approach-avoidance conflict of various kinds; the stutterer functions on the same principle. So the answer to why the stutterer gets stuck, at least on one level, is that he is in an approach-avoidance conflict; he is in a conflict between going ahead and holding back.

The Fear-Reduction Hypothesis. The occurrence of stuttering behavior reduces the fear that brought it about. This hypothesis has been developed to account for the release from or termination of the stuttering block. Thus the answer to the second question is that stuttering behavior itself actuates the moment of release. At the beginning of a block the stutterer is at point A; then he moves over to point B, the moment of release. Now how does he get from A to B? Why does he, for example, grimace, lower his eyes, jerk his head? Why does he take all of these curiously irrelevant but seemingly effective measures to produce a word? The fear-reduction hypothesis provides our answer to these questions.

In between A and B, the individual stutters; the stuttering reduces the fear, reduces the avoidance, reduces the holding back, so that he is now able to go on and finish the word. He is thus reinforced, his anxiety is reduced, and a vicious circle continues. Since he is constantly rewarded for stuttering, he keeps on keeping on. As long as the stutterer, in using some trick or device or crutch or bit of phony behavior, does succeed in producing the word, then he is going to continue those behaviors.

Now, in order to help the stutterer, we must deal with these twin features of the problem. We have to reduce the avoidance behavior and remove the reasons for it. We must break up the cycle of reinforcement.

An early experiment aimed at the reinforcement problem in stuttering, "The modification of stuttering through non-reinforcement" (Sheehan, 1951), may be cited at this point. The experimental procedure did not permit the stutterer to use his stuttering behavior as an instrumental act to produce the word. Instead of reading a passage "M-M-M-Many ancient peoples knew how to m-m-m-make iron," and leaving it like that, the stutterer would have to repeat each stuttered word until spoken once fluently. He would read thus: "M-M-M-Many m-m-many many ancient . . ." and so on throughout the passage. The last response, or the response closest to the termination of the sequence, then became a successful normal-speaking response. Therefore, instead of receiving their usual last-response reinforcement, stuttering responses were being systematically non-reinforced. Stuttering declined more rapidly under non-reinforcement than under a control condition, and the reduction was more lasting. In a sense, the study provided experimental support for one form of the technique of "cancellation."

In therapy we must deal somehow with the reinforcement aspect of stuttering. So long as the stutterer uses his tricks to get the words out, he is rewarded for this. Every time he stutters he is strengthening and learning his stuttering pattern. In therapy we must break up this inevitable reinforcement sequence.

In the treatment of stuttering, there is both an attitude aspect and a habit aspect: what is involved is partly a matter of feeling and partly a matter of motor behavior. Therefore what is indicated is partly a matter of psychotherapy and partly a matter of speech or action therapy. The concept of stuttering as approach-avoidance conflict provides logical direction for treatment and clarifies the psychotherapy-speech therapy relationship (Sheehan, 1954).

Spontaneous Recovery and Reinforcement

Along with the puzzle of the persistence of stuttering, we must account theoretically for the predominant nonpersistence of stuttering in the majority of cases in which the disorder begins. In a recent study, Sheehan and Martyn (1966) found that four out of five of those who begin to stutter recover spontaneously. Obviously, any learning theory which purports to account for reinforcement in 20 per cent of the cases must equally be able to account for failure of reinforcement in the 80 per cent of stutterers in whom the behavior disappears. Otherwise the theoretical account is incomplete and deficient.

Recovery may occur without therapy, with therapy, or in spite of it. It seems to involve a process similar to experimental extinction, for recovery from stuttering is now well established as a gradual process. Reliable and verifiable accounts of sudden cures just don't exist in the literature, although one may find here and there a recklessly distributed anecdote. Beginning with a well-known symposium of recovered stutterers in the 1957 American Speech and Hearing Association convention, accounts have agreed that recovery from stuttering occurs gradually over time. More recent reports by Wingate (1964), Shearer and Williams (1965), and Sheehan and Martyn (1966) have confirmed that recovery is typically gradual. This important finding supplies indirect evidence for learning theory interpretations of stuttering, and facilitates our viewing of recovery as probably an extinction process.

78

Is Stuttering a Unitary Disorder?

Stutterers are not a unique breed, a people apart. They range in personality structure as widely as do non-stutterers. As revealed by Rorschach, TAT, MMPI, and other personality assessment methods, there are stutterers who are hysteric, or compulsive, or elated, or depressed, or psychotic; but, to an astonishing degree, there are also stutterers who are normal—clinically normal. No single personality pattern exists for all stutterers, nor can stutterers be shown to differ from control groups of normal speakers.

The question of whether stuttering is a unitary disorder is a most important issue (Sheehan, 1958b, 1960). Stuttering is not a uniform problem, but a generic name for a whole group of disorders. Psychologically speaking, there seem to be several psychological or other subtypes of the disorder. Perhaps one reason that differences—personality, physiological, or physical—do not emerge in systematic comparisons of stutterers and non-stutterers is that the subtypes tend to cancel one another out, since the same subtypes may occur in the control group population.

In a survey of the Rorschach, TAT, and other projective tests (Sheehan, 1958a), essentially this conclusion was offered, viz., that one of the reasons there weren't more differences shown is that the group studies which statistical control necessitates produce a canceling or counterbalancing effect; the subtypes obscure one another. Berlin's doctoral research (1954) in which an attempt was made to isolate physiological and other subtypes, Frederick's studies at UCLA (1955) showing contrasting reactions to reward and punishment, Gregory's (1959, 1964a) studies, and Curry and Gregory's (1967) studies of the central neural auditory system support, to some degree, the possibility that subtypes of stutterers exist.

The possibility that there are identifiable psychological or other subtypes in stuttering deserves careful exploration (Sheehan, 1958a, 1960). A similar idea has recently been expressed by St. Onge (1963).

If there are several kinds of stutterers, each may call for a somewhat different approach to treatment. Moreover, to talk about *the* cause of *the* stuttering in a general sense is really nonsensical, for we must consider the type of stutterer in planning treatment.

Reinforcement in stuttering does not follow a single simple principle. Not every stutterer who persists does so on the same basis, nor in all

79

probability does every stutterer who fails to persist and becomes a recovered stutterer. The affects with which stutterers experience their moments of stuttering vary enormously among individuals, and are typically mixed. Along with release and tension-reduction for some stutterers in some of their blocks, there may be increases in shame, dejection, or guilt. Evidence for the foregoing statements may be found in the study by Sheehan, Cortese, and Hadley (1962), which should be compared with an earlier study by Wischner (1952a). An important conclusion of the Sheehan, Cortese, and Hadley study was that not all stutterers follow the same pattern of reinforcement, a view which should be underscored today.

For example, in comparing the effects of experimentally administered reward and punishment on stuttering, Frederick (cited earlier) found that while some subjects stuttered more frequently under punishment, others stuttered more frequently under reward for stuttering. He was able to differentiate these subgroups on the basis of the MMPI profiles. In the reward-increase group the D Scale was low, while the Hypochondriasis and Hysteria Scales were relatively elevated. Since anxiety was lower, it appeared that perhaps these were individuals whose stuttering behavior served a present neurotic need. They were not stuttering on a vicious circle basis, or on a self-perpetuation frustration basis. Rather, the anxiety was "bound in the symptom" in the classic Freudian sense.

Freud once proposed that neurotic symptoms are not problems in themselves, but are solutions to problems. A girl with a paralyzed arm, for example, had developed the paralysis in order not to take care of her invalid father toward whom she had an ambivalent attachment. She also expressed something in terms of what is called "organ language," a rather fascinating subtopic of the general problem of symptom formation. She wouldn't raise a hand to help her father! As Theodor Reik has noted, the unconscious is sometimes a very bad punster.

Here are other examples of organ language. A colleague of mine, who was being harassed by a rather aggressive younger colleague, developed a number of boils on his neck. Was somebody giving him, perhaps, a pain somewhere? Another man, in the presence of people he didn't like, would develop dermatitis. Was something getting under his skin? Still another individual, an aphasic, reacted to people he didn't like by getting a rectal itch. Now, the inference process here is fairly obvious. This then is the organ language component of neurotic symptoms.

Freud spoke of symptom formation as being a compromise between two forces which had entered into opposition—a precursor of ap-

80

proach-avoidance conflict. He proposed that the neurotic symptom or compromise bound the anxiety. The anxiety was contained, so that as long as the individual kept the symptom he would not experience the anxiety. If he gave up the symptom he would again suffer the anxiety unless he developed a new symptom.

Actually there is considerable doubt about the notion of symptom substitution, and no solid positive evidence in the literature. However, it fits in nicely with Freudian theory. If you view symptomatic behavior as a solution to a problem rather than as a problem, then of course the removal of the attempted symptomatic solution would not be a contribution in a positive direction. It would merely force the individual to devise a new solution.

The behavior called stuttering appears sufficiently complex, based upon the selective reinforcement of learned responses, so that it cannot be considered as a single symptom. Hence the interpretations of stuttering that can be made within the symptom-formation framework offered by Freud are fairly limited.

The locus of stuttering behavior is not simple, but varies from one individual to another and even within the same individual at different times and on different sounds. Thus you cannot consider stuttering as a direct expression of any kind of organ language, save that communication via speech is involved, and this at some point does require the vocal apparatus. But the "organs" involved in stuttering are so varied among stuttering patterns that no general organ meaning can be assigned to stuttering.

As the resultant of conflicting tendencies, for approach and for avoidance, for self-exposure and for self-concealment, stuttering behavior has an expressive aspect. Stuttering patterns themselves are the result of a long process of shaping, of continual modification through the irregular reinforcement of tricks and their eventual incorporation into the pattern. Yet the pattern is not just the chance product of random instrumental learning. All through his life the stutterer has been exercising choice in his selection of tricks or grimaces to cope with his fear. The choices are necessarily projective of the dynamics of the chooser and reflective of the interpersonal relationship out of which they emerge. Some stutterers are active and aggressive in their patterns; others are meek and acquiescent, nice guys finishing last verbally. With reference to the organ language component, each stutterer will in his pattern be expressing significant things about himself and his conceptions of his role. However, fairly direct, action-oriented treatment of the stutterer is still indicated. The stutterer changes through experience, through role-taking, and there appears to be little basis for fearing symptom substitution with the mixture of psychotherapy, speech therapy, and action therapy outlined below.

THERAPY SUMMARY

Principles of therapy for stutterers follow logically from the view of stuttering as a role conflict involving approach and avoidance behavior, as a false-role disorder. A number of these have already been indicated within the context of the theory presentation. Considerations of brevity limit the detail in which therapy can be covered here; however, here are, in summary fashion, some major guidelines for stuttering therapy:

1. Acceptance of self in the dual roles of stutterer and normal speaker, with renunciation of all false-role behavior.

2. Acceptance of responsibility for the behavior called stuttering. As an important step, realization by the stutterer that stuttering is something that he *does,* not something that happens to him.

3. Monitoring: continuous self-scrutiny by the stutterer of his on-going stuttering behavior. The stutterer conceals his problem not only from others but also from himself. Eye contact work is most important here, not only with others during moments of stuttering but also with self, using mirror and videotape feedback.

4. Initiative: as a part of reducing avoidance and strengthening approach tendencies, the seeking out of every opportunity to speak. The stutterer cannot afford to wait for situations to happen to him. He needs to be on the move, to work actively to eliminate avoidances, to build a set or attitude which readies him to greet each emerging speaking situation as an opportunity and a challenge; to seek, to tempt, to "court the fear." He needs to learn to use situations, rather than to let them use him.

5. Reducing the iceberg: As stated elsewhere (Sheehan, 1954, 1958b; Speech Foundation of America, 1960), the handicap of stuttering is like an iceberg, with the more significant portion lying beneath the surface. This is the portion—shame, guilt, attitudes of concealment, false-role—that must be brought above the surface, if recovery is ever to be complete or successful.

6. The role and the personality of the therapist: An aspect of therapy perhaps not sufficiently recognized by many therapists is the extent to which their own personalities shape the personalities of the stutterers

82

with whom they work (Sheehan, 1953b). Through the process of identification, many stutterers take on characteristics of their therapists, just as many children take on characteristics of their parents. The therapist influences the therapy process not only in formal orientation but also in many ways related directly to his own personality.

It is possible for the therapist to become concerned too deeply with procedures and methodologies, to forget that the most important variable in therapy, outside of the stutterer, is the therapist himself. Frequently his personal attributes are crucial in terms of therapy processes and outcome.

During the course of therapy the therapist enacts many different roles. As therapy progresses the function of the therapist may shift, so that he needs from time to time to pause, to re-evaluate, and occasionally to restructure his part in the therapeutic relationship. He needs to be flexible, to serve different functions at different stages.

Flexibility is an important element in therapeutic skill and success. Early in therapy, for example, the therapist must provide much support for the stutterer's venture of facing situations and people he has avoided, attacking old fears. At a later stage in therapy the therapist role may be quite different. He may need to help the stutterer accept and adjust to the consequences of his own improvement, or to teach socially constructive patterns of aggressiveness, or to help him explore new possibilities as he takes his part in a more fluent world.

VI

HAROLD L. LUPER

An Appraisal of Learning Theory

Concepts in Understanding and

Treating Stuttering in Children

PROBLEMS IN APPLYING CONCEPTS OF LEARNING THEORY TO STUTTERING

FEW CLINICIANS WOULD QUESTION THE STATEMENT that stuttering involves learned behavior to a very significant degree. Regardless of their views concerning the "original causes" of this condition, they see some learned behaviors in all stuttering problems. Most, I am sure, would also accept the fact that therapy involves learning; in fact, one might define therapy as a systematic learning situation for producing desirable changes in behavior.

Despite the obvious relationships between stuttering therapy and learning, there are some rather basic problems that make it difficult to apply principles or concepts of learning theory to stuttering and to

84

therapy for stutterers. Therefore, before attempting to show how therapy programs can utilize learning theory principles, I should like to discuss some of the factors which make such application difficult.

One reason stuttering is difficult to explain in learning theory terms is that the problem of stuttering is variable. Stuttering is manifested by a wide variety of symptoms. The old saying that no two stutterers are alike is doubtlessly true. We do not see the same exact speech behaviors, the same case history patterns, or the same degree of fear or embarrassment in any two people who stutter. Furthermore, the problem of stuttering in adults appears to be quite different from the problem bearing the same label in children.

Another aspect of stuttering that makes it difficult to study is its *intermittency*. Wendell Johnson once said that if measles were like stuttering, you could make a million dollars in a side show. "Just imagine," said Dr. Johnson, "how audiences would react if you had someone whose face turned bright red every few minutes and then, just as suddenly, returned to normal, only to break out again shortly with no obvious explanation." Stuttering is, indeed, very intermittent, and, even in the most severe stutterers, one can nevertheless find many times when they do not stutter. Despite the fact that one might predict in general those times when stuttering is more likely to occur, one still cannot predict exactly when or how a person will stutter. Stuttering is very transitory, very intermittent.

One of the major complicating factors in attempting to explain stuttering is the fact that it appears to consist of a series of *sequential* behaviors rather than being a discrete unit of behavior. Speech itself is a sequential act and when we examine stuttering "microscopically," it also appears to involve sequential behavior. When I first began trying to explain stuttering by learning theory concepts, I often utilized the following diagram:

(a) ^{S}threatening $\longrightarrow$ ^{R}stuttering
(b) ^{S}non-threatening $\longrightarrow$ ^{R}non-stuttering

It may be explained as follows:

(a) A stimulus to speak in a situation which the speaker perceives as threatening leads to a stuttering response; (b) a stimulus to speak in a situation which is perceived as non-threatening leads to a non-stuttering speech response.

Using this type of explanation, therapy was seen as aimed either at the left side of the diagram, that is, at changing the way the speaker viewed speaking situations; or at the right side, at changing the types of responses which the subject made in situations which were perceived as threatening.

There were several errors in this view of stuttering, but one of the most important was the error of oversimplicity. Stuttering is not a single discrete behavior in contrast to some other behavior that is labeled "non-stuttering." Nor is stuttering simply a collection of behaviors all elicited by the same stimulus. From a microscopic view of the events that transpire in any "moment" of stuttering, stuttering appears to be a long chain of stimulus-related responses. A greatly simplified, partial explanation of what happens in one "moment" of stuttering might look something like what we see in Table 3, though I am not sure how this would be

TABLE 3

"MICROSCOPIC" EXPLANATION (GREATLY SIMPLIFIED) OF ONE
INSTANCE OF ADVANCED STUTTERING

Time——→

Prestuttering Phase	Initiation Phase	Release Phase	Poststuttering Phase
1. Evaluation of potential difficulty	1. Search for possible avoidance device	1. Psychological defeat	1. Re-evaluation of listener response
2. Evaluation of probable listener's reaction	2. Trial attempt of avoidance device(s)	2. Tension build-up and struggle	2. Confirmation of personal inability to solve problem
	3. Evaluation of avoidance successfulness	3. Proprioceptive feedback punishment	3. Generalization of fear leading to reinforcement for avoidance and struggle behaviors
	4. Re-evaluation of situation	4. Confirmation of difficulty	
	5. Decision to make approach	5. Relief on termination	

diagramed using the common symbolization of learning theory. For example, let us assume that the speaker has perceived the utterance of the word at this particular time as being "dangerous." This may occur as he is talking, or before he begins to talk. Assuming that the speaker is an advanced stutterer who has already experienced a great deal of learning of this type, his next response is to begin to "sort" through his available devices for avoiding embarrassment and difficulty. He decides to try substituting a synonym, and, quickly, while he is still talking and moving closer to the point when he must utter the feared word, he comes up with a suitable substitute. As the stutterer starts to employ the avoidance behavior, he probably has an increase of what Mowrer (1960a) calls "hope." At the same time, the degree of tension in his speech musculature has been steadily increasing, so that even the substitute word may be distorted when uttered.

Assume for this illustration that, as is frequently the case in advanced stuttering, the attempt to avoid is unsuccessful. Either the speaker could not think of a suitable synonym, or he felt he would also stutter on it. So now the stutterer is confronted with making an attempt at this word which he perceives as being difficult. This point is shown in Table 3 as the Initiation Phase of the moment of stuttering. Again the stutterer is faced with a dilemma. Should he postpone the utterance or go ahead? He decides to postpone, but momentarily he is again back to the point where he must initiate the articulatory and phonatory movements necessary to begin the word. Assuming he has been in therapy, he may attempt a "loose contact," or he may try to force his way through this first initiation. Either one might result in a feeling of being blocked and being unable to continue talking. In this illustration, that is what happens.

In the Release Phase of the moment of stuttering which occurs while he is stuttering, the speaker still has some choices. He might try to struggle and force harder; he might be able to reduce the tension in the articulators consciously. Sooner or later the word is completed (unless our hypothetical stutterer gives up and finds some other way around his difficulty) and he is in the Poststuttering Phase. Here he may experience various emotions such as relief, embarrassment, guilt, or even pride if he felt he had endured an otherwise intolerable situation and if he felt his therapist or his friends would consider him more courageous for having done so. He may continue talking. He may speed up his speech to prove that he can still talk. He may even be able to maintain a certain degree of poise and return to a normal, less tense state of being.

The event I have outlined in Table 3 is actually the way one sophisticated stutterer recently analyzed one of his difficult situations. How can such a complicated sequence be described adequately? In fact, as I have labeled the diagram, even this explanation is greatly simplified and omits a great deal of information. Think of the number of different stimuli involved, the number of different responses made, and the numerous reinforcements that the speaker has received. An instance of stuttering is not just one response, but a series of responses, some being reinforced and others being extinguished.

The most nearly adequate way of dealing with this problem that I have seen thus far is that involving the concepts of "behavioral choice points," "sequential learning," and "response-correlated stimuli." Osgood (1953) uses these concepts in describing the sequential learning that takes place as a child learns to tie his shoes. In Osgood's explanation, the first stimulus in this sequential behavior might be a visual stimulus of looking down and seeing the shoe untied. The child's first response would be to pick up the shoestrings and pull them together. The response of picking up the strings creates certain proprioceptive feedback stimuli that, in turn, become stimuli for the next response, which would be, perhaps, to loop the strings. Such sequences of responses, where each response in a sequential act has within it certain stimuli that lead to the next response, are called response-correlated stimuli. In sequential learnings, Osgood feels that there are important behavioral choice points—points in time where one stimulus sets off a whole series of other stimuli and responses.

I believe that Osgood's explanation of sequential learning is very applicable to the problem of stuttering. A person in the act of stuttering encounters a large number of behavioral choice points. He may come up to a word and debate over whether to avoid it or to plunge ahead and attempt to use it (an approach-avoidance conflict). Once he has made one response, other stimuli and responses are set off, each having the potential of being reinforced. In a short time, he comes to another behavioral choice point—another place where he sees an option to his behavior—and again he sets off a chain of response-correlated stimuli.

As I have been trying to point out, stuttering is an extremely difficult kind of behavior to describe in learning theory concepts. It is very intermittent, it varies a great deal from one individual to another, and it appears to be a type of sequential behavior, consisting of many stimuli and many responses, rather than an isolated event. We have a very hard time in the field of speech pathology in agreeing on single instances of stuttering. Experimental studies of learning, on the other hand, tend to involve relatively simple behaviors in situations where the important variables are fairly easy to control. To explain stuttering in traditional S-R terms is to oversimplify it. As I said earlier, I feel quite strongly that the problem called stuttering involves a great deal of what is commonly referred to as learning, but I do not believe that the psychology of learning has yet developed concepts that can give more than a rough approximation of the learning involved in stuttering. The fault may be the clinicians—I am not sure. The problem may lie in their inability to define the problem of stuttering in behavioral terms that can be utilized effectively in studies of learning.

In order that the reader may understand better what I am referring to when I use the terms "stuttering," "stuttering behavior," or "stuttering problem," let me briefly define my use of these words. The term "stuttering problem" is, for me, the broadest term in the group. As I normally use it, it refers to all of the speech and non-speech behaviors associated with the speaker's feeling that he cannot talk as spontaneously as he desires. The term "stuttering behavior" refers to any single act the person performs in trying to speak or to avoid speaking when he feels he will stutter. My definition of the single word "stuttering" is much more specific and needs some amplification.

As I see it, stuttering is an involuntary delay in timing or an audible distortion in the utterance of speech sounds due to excessive pressure in the emission of air or excessive force in the articulatory and phonotary contacts necessary to emit a speech sound. In other words, stuttering is not simply disfluent speech. Many disfluencies are "normal" and, as Johnson's studies have pointed up, stuttering speech is sometimes more fluent than non-stuttering speech. Nor is stuttering simply a greater than normal amount of tension in the speech musculature; but it is excess tension that is great enough to produce an abnormal delay or an audible distortion of the speech output.

Perhaps another way to say this is that stuttering results when the speaker is unable to cope with excess muscular tension in the speech mechanism. For example, in faked or pseudo-stuttering, a speaker can greatly increase the tension in the speech musculature and still have the ability to cope with it. A stutterer who has learned to "fake" stuttering can frequently exhibit a speech pattern that sounds almost identical to his "real" stuttering. Such a person will often say that he was not stuttering (he usually says "that wasn't a real one"). Apparently the speaker's perception of his ability to cope with the excess tension—to continue talking without an abnormal delay in timing or an audible distortion of the speech output—is the main determinant of whether he calls the stuttering real or faked.

Figure 19 presents another view of my current concept of stuttering. This figure attempts to explain two major parameters of the problem of stuttering. Line A illustrates the highly variable degree of tension in the speech musculature that occurs from moment to moment in any speaker. Line B represents a similar variation in another speaker. The horizontal

90

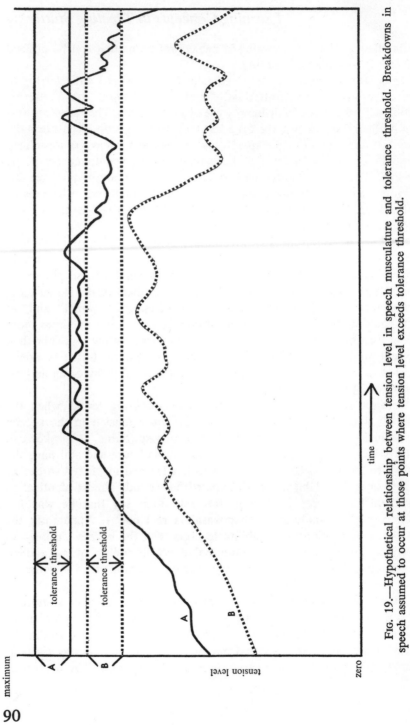

Fig. 19.—Hypothetical relationship between tension level in speech musculature and tolerance threshold. Breakdowns in speech assumed to occur at those points where tension level exceeds tolerance threshold.

lines near the top of the figure represent the less variable *capacity* of the individual to continue talking without abnormal delays in timing or audible distortions in the speech output. As I envision the problem, stuttering would occur when the individual's degree of tension in the speech musculature exceeds his tolerance threshold for withstanding excess tension. At the point where this occurs, the individual is unable to continue talking without an abnormal delay in timing or an audible distortion of speech. This figure also attempts to illustrate that different individuals have different degrees of tension as they speak, and that some can withstand greater tension without speech "breaking down" than can others (B would not stutter; see Fig. 19).

I would assume that the tolerance threshold is affected by such factors as the stability of the individual's language skills, his concept of himself as a speaker, and his general physical and emotional state. For example, we find more frequent speech breakdowns (repetitions, hesitations, etc.) among young children whose language skills are still not fully developed than among adults. The tension level, on the other hand, is affected by such things as approach-avoidance conflicts (Sheehan, 1954), fears of speaking, general bodily tension, and the like. In other words, speech is an activity that requires rapid, smooth adjustments in order to proceed at a normal rate and with a pleasant voice. When the tension in the speech musculature exceeds an individual's tolerance level, he exhibits abnormal delays in the timing of his articulatory contacts and has audible distortions in speech output as a result.

Probably the most important phenomenon to be explained in stuttering is why some speakers have more of these abnormal delays in timing and audible distortions of speech than others. It is quite possible that learning theory cannot explain this phenomenon. Note that my explanation of tension and tolerance level did not rely solely on principles or concepts from the field of psychology of learning.

SOME ASSUMPTIONS ABOUT STUTTERING AND THE LEARNING OF STUTTERING

In analyzing the development of stuttering in children and adults, one is confronted with a question concerning *how a speaker learns* the complex behaviors that characteristically are a part of stuttering. From my observations of stutterers and from the literature in speech development, stuttering, and the psychology of learning, I would make the following assumptions concerning the learning of stuttering:

1. *Disfluencies in speech result from many factors.* In my earlier discussion of tension and tolerance threshold levels and stuttering, I mentioned some of the factors that lead to abnormal disfluencies. Probably the largest number of speech disfluencies are within the normal range of speaking behavior, and the conditions leading to these normal disfluencies must be almost infinite in number.

2. *Disfluent speech, in itself, is not necessarily punishing.* Stating this differently, the act of being disfluent is frequently not bothersome either to the speaker or to the listener. Disfluent speech is sometimes used purposefully to convey some of the prosodic aspects of speech. Disfluent speech may be related to the cognitive processes of the speaker. It may even occur in abnormal form, yet go unnoticed due to concentration upon the content of the communication. The point being made here is not that disfluent speech *cannot* be punishing, but that there is nothing inherently punitive about speech that lacks fluency.

3. *The occurrence of disfluencies may be unpleasant, that is, punishing, if followed by "negative" social reinforcement.* By negative social reinforcement I refer to events such as parental reprimanding or loss of listener attention. Since all speech therapists are very much aware of the problems that can be caused by parental overreaction to a child's disfluencies, I do not believe I need to amplify this point.

4. *Disfluent speech that is accompanied by excess tension in the speech musculature is unpleasant and, therefore, punishing, because it interferes with communication and creates unpleasant kinesthetic and acoustic feedback.* Earlier, I stated the assumption that disfluent speech was not necessarily punishing. The assumption was also made that negative social feedback could serve to make the act of being disfluent a punishing event. The present statement is intended to make clear still a different condition for a child to associate disfluency with punishment. In this statement, I assume that excess tension in the speech musculature is unpleasant because it tends to make the act of speaking more difficult and at the same time it provides acoustic and kinesthetic feedback which the speaker does not enjoy.

5. *Increased tension that the individual feels capable of handling is not as punishing as increased tension with which the individual feels he cannot cope.* There is more punishment attached to a situation where the individual feels he does not have control over his own behavior. I am convinced that this is one of the most important aspects of therapy for advanced stutterers. The person who feels he has no control over his stuttering fears it more than one who has learned he can modify his

speech behavior even though he is experiencing increased tension. The so-called modification techniques, such as loose contacts, frequently provide the stutterer with a way to cope with his problem. Once he feels he can do something to change his stuttering, the event of feeling blocked becomes less punishing.

6. *The frequent occurrence of unpleasantness with disfluencies increases the speaker's expectation of unpleasantness in the same situation at later times.* This assumption also needs little amplification. It is an example of what Mowrer (1960a) would call "once-always generalization," wherein the speaker generalizes from past to future experiences. As Mowrer points out, all learning can be thought of as "once-always generalization."

7. *The frequent occurrence of unpleasantness with disfluencies increases the speaker's expectation that he will have difficulty in other speaking situations.* This, of course, is just another way of saying that children will generalize the speech difficulties they have in one situation to other situations which they perceive as being similar. Figure 20 illustrates the principle of generalization of learning. In this particular example, taken from a classical study of conditioning, four groups of pigeons were conditioned to respond to four different colors. The wave lengths of the colors are shown on the abscissa of Figure 20. For example, one group was reinforced (received food) only when a color having a wavelength of 530 mμ (I believe that was green) could be seen just above the opening that dispensed the food. Another group was reinforced only when a color having a wavelength of 550 mμ was visible, and so forth. The number of times the pigeons responded is shown by the height of the curve (the ordinate of Fig. 20). This study by Guttman and Kalish (1956) demonstrates quite clearly that when an organism is reinforced for responding to one stimulus, he tends to respond to other stimuli in much the same way (assuming that he sees a similarity between the other stimuli and the one for which he is being reinforced). Furthermore, the organism's responses are related to the degree of similarity between the original stimulus and the others. I know of no reason to expect children to be much different from these pigeons or from any other organism that has been studied. If some kind of punishment occurs frequently when the child is disfluent in one situation, he would tend to expect unpleasantness to occur in other situations in which he is disfluent.

8. *The more frequently one feels incapable of coping with excess tension, the more likely he is to resort to struggle behavior, to attempt to*

93

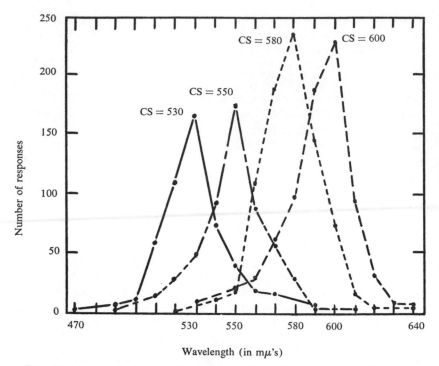

FIG. 20.—Generalization gradients reported by Guttman and Kalish (1956, p. 83).

avoid the unpleasantness, and to assume he is generally incapable of talking correctly. The point here is that the feeling of being unable to cope with the excess tension leads to the habitual struggle behaviors and avoidances and to a generalized self-concept of being an inadequate speaker.

9. *Word and situation fears develop most readily when frequent difficulty is experienced on the same word or in the same situation and when the individual is very aware of having difficulty.* We would expect, for example, that difficult words which are used frequently would become more feared than words on which the speaker might experience as much actual speech difficulty, but which occur less often in his communicative experiences. We would also expect that the stuttering utterance of a word in a highly embarrassing situation would be more likely to lead to generalization of word fears than stuttering of equal severity that occurs in a situation where the speaker is not overly aware of his difficulty. For

example, many stutterers report that they have more difficulty saying their name than saying other words. Perhaps a speaker finds it particularly embarrassing to be hesitant in responding when someone asks his name, and, therefore, he is highly aware of his difficulty at this time.

10. *Generalization of fears to other words is more likely to occur when there is phonetic, semantic, or orthographic similarity to the other words.* This is another way of saying that word fears will generalize to those words that the speaker views as similar. If he is a nonreader, one would not expect much orthographic generalization. On the other hand, if he is a person who has more difficulty when reading aloud, one would predict generalization on an orthographic basis because the stutterer has probably developed a habit of looking at the printed word to see if it has one of his "hard" sounds in it. Most therapists have probably worked with stutterers who indicated they could not say words beginning with the letter *f*, yet showed no fear of words beginning with the letters *ph*.

11. *A general self-concept of being handicapped is most likely to occur when the speech difficulty is long term and widespread, and when the instances of stuttering are magnified.* This is simply to say that the longer the person has abnormal disfluencies, or the more generalized his difficulties are in terms of words and situations, or the more these are brought to his attention in some way, then the more likely he is to develop a self-concept of being different—of being handicapped. His difficulties may be magnified by listener reaction or by self-imposed penalties, such as frustration. One of the more common ways to magnify the problem is to label the speaker a stutterer. It may also be magnified by subconscious psychological reasons for being dependent or for failing. Regardless of how it occurs, magnification of the disfluency increases the probability that the speaker will generalize from a self-concept of "I am a person who sometimes has difficulty speaking" to "I am a handicapped person."

I have discussed some of the difficulties in applying traditional learning theory concepts to stuttering and have made some assumptions regarding the learning of stuttering. The variability, transitory intermittency, and sequential form of stuttering indicate that this is a highly complex behavior which is hard to "catch" and "pin down" for study. According to my current view of stuttering, a suitable explanation of the problem must include terms such as "involuntary," "excess pressure," and "tension-tolerance threshold"—terms which do not readily lend themselves to learning theory explanations. Despite my inability to make a clear-cut case for explaining stuttering completely in learning theory terms, there seems to be little question that much learning does take place in the development of stuttering. I attempted to specify some of the assumptions that I make in regard to the learning that takes place in the problem of stuttering. I shall now deal with therapy and see how principles of learning can apply to the modification or elimination of stuttering behaviors.

Goals of the Therapist for Children Who Stutter

When therapy is viewed as a learning experience, the therapist's role resembles that of the experimenter in a learning experiment. The therapist, like the experimenter, hopes to control to some extent stimuli and reinforcements with the eventual aim of changing certain parts of the learner's behavior. Both the experimenter and the therapist must decide beforehand on the endpoint—the target—of the learning experience so that they will know when and how to reinforce the subject's responses. If I were to name some of the more important goals for the therapy learning experience, they would probably include the following:

1. To decrease the frequency of the type of speech responses that lead to negative reinforcement.[1]

2. To decrease the number of negative reinforcements the child receives when he is disfluent.

3. To prevent the child from developing inappropriate methods for solving his problems.

4. To prevent the child from making harmful generalizations about his difficulty.

Looking at these goals, it will be noted that the first goal implies that the therapist has a responsibility to help the child modify the speech behavior itself, if we assume that disfluent speech accompanied by excess tension is likely to lead to negative reinforcement. Based on the further assumption that some speech disfluencies are not punishing, one task in therapy might be to reinforce disfluencies that are less tense, less abnor-

1. Editor's note: The author is using negative reinforcement to mean punishment; it is used in this way by many learning theorists. However, Skinner refers to the removal of punishment as negative reinforcement.

mal, less likely to lead to negative reinforcement. The therapist should be able to "shape" the child's responses by gradually raising the requirement for reinforcement—first reinforcing any response that is less tense than the average, then gradually raising the standards so that he reinforces only the "normal" disfluency. Incidentally, in order to help the child produce more "non-tense" responses (which can then be reinforced), the therapist may need to utilize some modification techniques, such as loose contacts.

The second goal requires that the therapist work with people other than the child who stutters. If the number of negative reinforcements the child receives in any situation other than a one-to-one therapy relationship is to be reduced, the therapist will have to work with those people in the child's environment who are most likely to be able to provide reinforcements. This is not saying anything new. For years, most therapists have worked with parents in the attempt to help them change their administration of reinforcements. They have been asked not to label, not to call attention to—in other words, not to punish—the child's disfluencies. Perhaps therapists could improve their techniques in this direction if they looked more closely at the learning problem involved on the part of the parents.

It has long been pointed out by speech pathologists that a large part of the problem of stuttering appears to be due to the stutterer's attempts to avoid the stuttering. Stating this in a different way, the stutterer appears to be using inappropriate methods for solving the problem of feeling "blocked." The third objective relates to this point. Again, perhaps the principles of shaping behavior can be employed. When a child uses a "trick" to get around a hard word, he is penalized in some way; when he goes directly into the hard word and hangs on to it without struggling or forcing, the therapist rewards him.

One of the major differences between younger, beginning stutterers and older, advanced stutterers seems to be the extent to which they generalize their difficulties. Everyone has difficulty talking at times; some children generalize this to the point where they expect to have trouble most of the time. The advanced stutterer tends to generalize his difficulty in speech to his ability in other skills and begins to feel that he is "inferior" or "handicapped" in all ways. One objective of therapy then is to prevent the child from making these harmful generalizations. This, perhaps, is the type of learning that is hardest to control in stuttering therapy. Perhaps we can help by having parents, teachers, and others praise the child for his accomplishments in other skills. It may be

97

possible to arrange the child's participation in various situations so that he has more "positive speaking experiences."

Extinction and Counterconditioning

I have listed some of the more important objectives of the learning situation in stuttering. Does the psychology of learning offer any clues as to how to proceed in helping the stutterer eliminate undesirable responses? I believe there are two concepts from the psychology of learning that might be useful. One of these is the process called *extinction;* the other bears the name of *counterconditioning.* Briefly defined, extinction refers to a weakening in the tendency to produce a response following nonreinforcement. If, on the other hand, the subject produces a response to a stimulus, but is provided the opposite kind of reinforcement (positive *vs.* negative rewards), this is counterconditioning.

How can these two concepts be applied to stuttering therapy? As part of a therapy session with an eleven-year-old girl who stuttered, I asked her to respond to one of my questions with the word *bullet.* She avoided this by saying, "I can't say that word." When I encouraged her to try it anyway, she stuttered rather severely on the "b" sound at the beginning of the word. Analyzing this in learning terminology, one could say that the stimulus was the expectation of stuttering and the response was the increased tension on the lips that made the utterance of the word difficult. Although she stuttered when she tried it, she did not receive any negative social feedback—that is, no adverse listener reactions from me. I asked her to continue saying the word and after a few trials she no longer stuttered. In speech therapy, this is called "stuttering adaptation"; in psychology of learning, it is known as extinction. In other words, the tendency for her to tighten up her lips as she starts to say the word "bullet" has been decreased because she has continued to make the same response but without receiving any negative reinforcement. An interesting question here is what has been extinguished—the fear of stuttering, the response of tightening up her lips, or both?

Continuing with applications of the concept of extinction to stuttering therapy, one might well ask if the extinction will be permanent or temporary? The results of extinction studies would lead to the prediction that the extinction process just described would be only temporary—that many, many more extinction trials would be necessary to completely eliminate the response of tightening up when she started to say the word "bullet." In the case of this girl, that is what occurred. When I returned to the same question after having her answer other questions, she would again tighten up and stutter. Extinction is a useful process to employ in therapy—therapists can have stutterers re-enter their hard situations, say again their hard words, or practice again their undesirable secondary responses; and if they can prevent reinforcement of their responses, the responses would probably be eliminated after a sufficient number of trials. However, extinction might be very slow and inefficient.

Why is extinction sometimes inefficient? First, it is known that if a response is originally learned on a partial reinforcement schedule, extinction will be much slower than if it were learned on a regular reinforcement basis. As Shames and Sherrick (1963) point out, stuttering is probably reinforced on a highly irregular schedule. Parents do not always react negatively to a child's stuttering. Such irregularity in original reinforcement makes extinction much slower. Secondly, extinction operates by nonreinforcement. I believe it is quite likely that even though the therapist in the case mentioned above withheld negative social reinforcement, the child experienced some negative proprioceptive or auditory self-reinforcement when she stuttered. This self-reinforcement would tend to work against the extinction process and thus make it slower and less efficient.

It appears then that something more than extinction is needed if stuttering responses are to be eliminated in any reasonable length of time. Perhaps the second process for eliminating responses—the process of counterconditioning—can be of help. To illustrate counterconditioning, let me return to the eleven-year-old girl. Suppose that instead of just remaining neutral when the child stuttered on the word "bullet," I praised her for making an attempt on the word. The child then would begin to receive positive reinforcement for attempting the word, rather than negative reinforcement or nonreinforcement for stuttering. Before counterconditioning, saying the feared word led to stuttering and negative self or social reinforcement. In counterconditioning, the saying of the word leads to the therapist's praise, so, therefore, it is rewarding.

Note also that the counterconditioning can be (and frequently is) interpreted in a different way. Counterconditioning is frequently thought to occur because a response that is incompatible with the previously conditioned response is rewarded. In the case of the girl, two undesirable responses can be seen—the avoidance of saying the word and tensing up the articulators; and two desirable responses (from the therapist's viewpoint)—making a normal approach response to saying the word and saying it with relaxed articulators. In the counterconditioning example, the therapist praised the child for approaching the feared word (this is

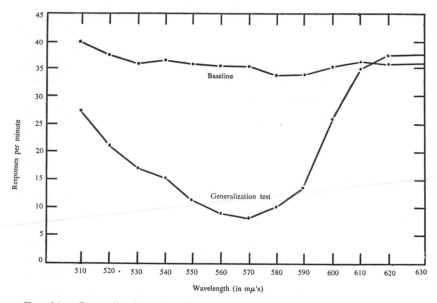

FIG. 21.—Generalization of extinction obtained by Honig (1961). Extinction trials were to stimulus of 570 mμ.

incompatible with avoiding it) and for using a loose contact (incompatible with tensing up the articulators). Regardless of how we interpret it, counterconditioning appears to be more effective than straight extinction for the elimination of undesired stuttering responses.

With the complex learning that has already taken place by the time the therapist sees a child in therapy, the task of helping the child unlearn his stuttering responses, with either extinction, counterconditioning, or both, appears to be extremely long and laborious. Stutterers have so many feared words, so many feared situations, so many avoidance and struggle behaviors, that it might take the rest of the child's lifetime to extinguish all of the undesirable stuttering responses.

Does learning theory have any suggestions for shortening this process? I believe so. Returning to the concept of generalization, shown in Figure 21 is a summary of the results of an extinction study using pigeons conducted by Honig (1961). In Honig's study, the pigeons were first reinforced for pecking to a large number of different stimuli—in this case, different colors. The baseline near the top of the graph represents the number of responses the pigeons were making after this first, condi-

100

tioning part of the study. As can be seen from the baseline curve, the pigeons made an approximately equal number of responses to all stimuli.

In the second part of Honig's study, the experimenter withheld reinforcement when a color having a wave length of 570 mμ (pure green) was displayed above the food-dispensing opening. Reinforcement was continued for all other colors. The lower curve in Figure 21 shows the results. Notice that not only was there a marked reduction in responses to the 570 mμ wavelength–the nonreinforced wavelength–but that fewer responses occurred to other wavelengths, particularly to those stimuli that were most similar to the nonreinforced stimulus. In other words, this lower curve illustrates generalization of extinction.

Applying generalization of extinction to stuttering therapy, it might be said that the extinction or counterconditioning done in therapy may be expected to spread to other *situations that are similar*. And if the new learning or unlearning is to have more effect, the child must experience this reduced stuttering in as many situations as possible. This explains, perhaps, why much of therapy is ineffective. Therapists tend to work with children in one situation only—in the therapy room. All therapists have had children whose stuttering has been reduced after a few sessions. A little of this may be expected to transfer to other situations— primarily to those situations that are quite similar to the therapy setting. But if this effect is to spread, the child must continue to make the same kind of responses in a wide variety of situations and continue to get the same kind of reinforcement that he has been getting in therapy.

How can therapists do this? They can train parents and teachers to react somewhat the same as they do, that is, to stop punishing the stuttering behavior by parental reprimands but to reward a stutterer's attempts to talk, particularly when he talks with reduced tension. The therapist can see to it that the child has many pleasurable speaking experiences. In terms of counterconditioning, the therapist can have him re-enter the same situation where he did have fear and incorporate some fun into it. It often helps, for example, to enroll a child in a creative dramatics class, if he can enjoy speaking before a small group. It might be appropriate to spend part of the time having the child read, part of the time having him recite from memory, and part of the time taking him into hard situations, instead of spending all of the time carrying on a conversation with him in the therapy room, as I have seen a few therapists do. In therapy, then, one can eliminate undesirable responses and teach new responses by proper use of extinction, counterconditioning, and generalization.

Barriers to Successful Control of the Learning Situation

Thus, certain concepts from the psychology of learning appear useful in working with stutterers. Perhaps, though, some may feel the explanations given above were too easy. Despite our knowledge of learning principles, it is frequently difficult to manipulate all of the important factors for the relearning that is involved in therapy. Let me mention a few of the important barriers to successful adaptation of learning principles in stuttering therapy.

One barrier is the therapist's inability to control the total learning situation. As indicated earlier, stuttering is reinforced on a highly variable schedule. If stutterers were punished every time they stuttered or every time they attempted to speak, the problem would be quite different than it is, where most of the stutterer's speaking experiences tend to be successful and only a small percentage of them are punishing.

Secondly, it is quite difficult to control all of the reinforcers in the environment. When one asks what reinforces the stuttering or reinforces the responses that are incompatible with stuttering, he comes up with a fairly large list. It has been hypothesized by Wischner (1950) and by Sheehan (1953a) that fear-reduction is the reinforcing agent in stuttering. This hypothesis has its roots in some of the earlier work by Mowrer (1939), Dollard and Miller (1950), and in the earlier drive-reduction theory of Hull (1943). According to the fear-reduction hypothesis in stuttering, the fear of uttering a word elicits the stuttering responses; and the reduction of fear that occurs upon the completion of the utterance of the feared word reinforces the behaviors that occurred just prior to the completion of the word.

Figure 22 illustrates the theoretical relationship between anxiety reduction and reinforcement. In looking at this graph, the points labeled "A," "B," and "C" refer to points in time during the stutterer's attempt to say a feared word. The height of the curve illustrates the relative degree of reinforcement given to the behaviors occurring at those points. Thus, the behaviors that occur closer in time to the point of reinforcement are theoretically reinforced more than those that occur earlier. This is known as the goal gradient hypothesis.

To take a hypothetical situation, assume that at point "A" the stutterer stopped and started over, at point "B" blinked his eyes, and at point "C," he jerked his head. Shortly thereafter the "blocked" word was emitted and the stutterer experienced a feeling of relief (fear-reduction) which reinforced the head jerk most and the retrial least.

102

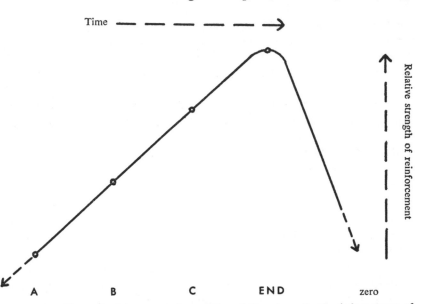

Fɪɢ. 22.—Theoretical representation of the relative strength of reinforcement of behaviors occurring at different temporal degrees of remoteness from the completion of the stuttering act (after Luper, 1956).

There is one aspect of this that has not yet been mentioned. If the avoidance behavior (such as the stopping and starting over) is successful in delaying the feared word, it is partially rewarding even if it does not completely avoid the feared word. Since any retrial will delay the utterance of a word, all would be expected to have some reward value. This may explain why stutterers will continue to use avoidance patterns even though the avoidances do not appear to help them in avoiding the feared situation or feared word.

If fear-reduction does reinforce the undesirable behaviors, what can the therapist do to surmount this barrier? There would appear to be three main methods. One would be to work toward changing the basic stimulus (fear) that leads to the stuttering responses. A second method for surmounting this barrier would be to provide other reinforcements that would compete with the reinforcement that comes from anxiety-reduction. And the third would be to delay the completion of the word until other, more desirable, responses were made. For example, the therapist might provide other reinforcements in the form of praise or might delay the completion of the word by use of a technique such as

103

"pull-out," in which the stutterer is asked to see if he can decrease the tension in the articulators before saying the remainder of the word. Since the voluntary reduction of tension comes last, it should be reinforced more than the undesirable responses, such as the head jerks or eye blinks.

Returning to the problem of being unable to control all of the important reinforcers of the child's stuttering, it can be seen that there are many reinforcers not under the therapist's control. The child's own feelings of relief when he avoids a word without the therapist's knowledge, the proprioceptive and auditory sensations he receives when he stutters or almost stutters, the various listener reactions from peers, parents, teachers, and so forth, all constitute important reinforcers for the child's stuttering or his attempts to speak. Most of these cannot be manipulated very easily by the therapist, and, therefore, make the task of helping the child learn new responses more difficult.

One of the problems in therapy is being unable to provide the proper reinforcement at the proper time. Recently, I was working with a stutterer, and, in the middle of a long utterance, he did the best job I had ever seen him do in terms of working his way through a stuttered word without abnormality. I should have reinforced him right at the moment, but I did not see an easy way to do it without interfering with his communication. That is a rather simple illustration of the problem of providing the proper reinforcement at the proper time. Most therapists see their stutterers only an hour or so each week. Think of the number of times the stutterers are making responses that need to be reinforced when they are not in therapy.

Another barrier to successful therapy is the difficulty in determining the amount and type of learning that has already taken place. With an older stutterer, the therapist sometimes gains a relatively good idea by talking to him of how much fear he has learned and what kinds of avoidances he has habituated. When working with children, however, the therapist is forced to guess a lot of this. One hesitates to come out and ask the child if he fears stuttering or talking because one does not want to put ideas into his head that are not already there.

Finally, I will mention one last barrier to the successful control of the learning situation in stuttering. This is the difficulty in motivating clients to want strongly enough to change so that they are willing to undergo temporary hardship. How does the therapist encourage a young stutterer to carry out the necessary tasks so that he can then reinforce the desirable responses? I am inclined to think that this is one of the biggest problems in public school therapy. Children do not always come in as motivated as adults do when they voluntarily request therapy. Young children tend to be so sensitive about their problem that they are unwilling to take the steps that are necessary to make responses that can be reinforced. For example, how can one reinforce a less tense articulatory contact when the child refuses to try the word? This barrier, although difficult, is not insurmountable. From operant conditioning studies, it is known that it is possible to lead a subject to make the desirable response by reinforcing those responses that approximate the desired goal. The therapist might first reward the child for coming to therapy. Later, the same child would be reinforced only if he talked. After this, he would be reinforced only for being willing to attempt his feared words, and, finally, reinforcement might be withheld unless he used a light articulatory contact.

Preventing Undesirable Responses

Most of the therapy mentioned so far refers to what might be done with the person who has already learned to fear or who has already developed inappropriate struggle and avoidance behaviors. How is the learning situation different when working with children whose disfluencies, avoidances, and struggles have not yet reached habit strength? First of all, the therapist is probably going to be working more on the stimulus end of the S-R bond than on the response end. As has been pointed out by Shames and Sherrick (1963), the therapist should attempt to prevent children from reacting to disfluencies as a discriminative class of stimuli. All individuals make both fluent and disfluent speech responses. Children make proportionately more disfluent responses than do adults. Unless something stands out to make the child react to his disfluent speech responses in some way different from his fluent behaviors, he should not notice them as being different and should not develop fears and struggle behaviors in response to his disfluencies. So what should be done? Tell parents not to call the disfluencies to the child's attention. All therapists have probably made such suggestions, and in terms of learning principles, they appear to be helpful.

In what other ways can the therapist work with the child who has not yet learned fear and habitual stuttering behaviors? He must try to help the parents decide what events make the child tense up more and thus increase the probability of his making disfluent speech responses. Then we can see what can be done to alter these situations. Does this make sense in terms of learning theory? Yes, if one assumes that the more disfluent the child is, the greater are his opportunities to receive punishment and thus begin to fear being disfluent.

For example, suppose that a child has many more disfluencies when reading aloud than in other speaking situations. The task then becomes one of trying to find out why this situation is more difficult for him. Perhaps he is having difficulty learning to read and thus becomes unsure of himself and hesitates because he is unsure. In this instance, the best therapy for him might be to provide some remedial reading instruction. On the other hand, it may be that parents or others are putting undue pressure on the child to read rapidly. The task here becomes one of changing the external pressure which the child is feeling.

SUMMARY

I have been dealing with the problem of applying principles of learning to stuttering and to stuttering therapy. As I indicated, it appears to me that the psychology of learning can be utilized to explain a great deal—but not all—of the questions about the origin and development of stuttering. There are many observed facts about stuttering that are difficult to explain in learning terms. For example, how can learning theory explain the large difference in incidence of the problem between males and females? Why does stuttering so rarely begin in adulthood? How can learning theory explain the relative infrequency of stuttering in the total speech output of the confirmed stutterer? These are just a few of the questions which to me are not answered satisfactorily by learning theory. On the other hand, learning theory concepts do not appear to conflict with other theories of the etiology of stuttering. Even if the original instigator of stuttering is of an emotional or physical nature, learning still has to take place for the fears, avoidances, and struggle behaviors to spread to the large variety of sounds and speaking situations which are characteristic of the problem in its advanced stages. The psychology of learning helps us to understand and to predict the learning that takes place in stuttering.

From a therapy standpoint, work with stutterers would appear to be helped by an understanding of principles of learning. Although stuttering is a highly complex behavior that is difficult to control in a systematic fashion, an understanding of the principles of learning should help the therapist in planning therapy, in understanding why certain procedures are sometimes successful, and in forming some testable hypotheses about the elimination of the problem.

VII

HUGO H. GREGORY

Applications of Learning Theory

Concepts in the Management of

Stuttering

THE PRIMARY PURPOSE OF THIS SYMPOSIUM has been to evaluate the concept of stuttering as a persistent, unadaptive habit that has been learned and to appraise the usefulness of learning theory principles in the treatment of the disorder. My specific purpose is to point out, discuss, and evaluate the applications of principles of learning in the management of stuttering at various stages of development and in some differing therapeutic settings.

Before getting into a consideration of some of these applications, I should like to make a few general statements pertaining to my present point of view about stuttering. It will be recalled that Johnson referred to "the conditions that tend to occasion increased nonfluency in young children" (Johnson, 1956, p. 294). The specific conditions he mentioned, with perhaps one exception (the situation in which the child is telling things for which he does not have adequate vocabulary), are related most directly to the child's interaction with the environment. Other examples are speaking to unresponsive listeners and speaking in competition with others. Situations of this type might be viewed as hazards to fluency. Rutherford (1963) has been interested in the way in which disruptions in the flow of speech might be occasioned by subtle expressive language deficits, such as the inability to call up a needed word. We have observed, at Northwestern, that children who have had expressive language problems go through periods of increased disfluency as the condition improves. Some clinical cases in which stuttering, or possible stuttering, is the focal question in our evaluation have been found to have minimal problems of motor patterning for the production of speech or difficulty related to auditory memory span.

I should like to call attention to an opinion, frequently stated during the last fifteen years, that research studies concerning group differences between stutterers and non-stutterers have tended to conceal etiological factors which could be of significance in certain stutterers. The ideas of "contributing factors which combine in various ways to produce stuttering," "different types of stutterers," or "different avenues to becoming a stutterer" seem to have gained increasing attention. Historically, Van Riper (1947, 1954, 1963) has been associated with this viewpoint. In recent years, Bloodstein (1958), in his anticipatory struggle hypothesis, appears to adhere to a multiple origin concept. Bloodstein makes reference to clinical evidence in pointing out that a child may come to have the conviction that speech demands unusual precaution when certain conditions exist: (1) If he is retarded in language development, has defective articulation, shows cluttering, has reading difficulty, or shows any kind of verbal ineptness; (2) if he is subjected to excessive parental demands for more adequate speech; and (3) if he has certain personality traits, for example, the tendency to be unusually sensitive or fearful, which may render him more vulnerable.

The procedures which I will present are based on a general theoretical conception that learned behavior patterns are of great significance in the problem of stuttering, but that certain conditions, such as individual differences (which are perhaps physical), influence in an important way the development of fluency in speech. Certain physical, as well as environmental, variables can occasion more disfluency and possibly qualitatively different types of disfluency; certainly these should be evaluated carefully and given consideration in the treatment of a stuttering problem.

In the young child (usually three to six years of age) speech clinicians have hoped to prevent or minimize the development of anxiety about speech as a learned source of drive. Or, to use the terminology of another school of learning (operant conditioning), clinicians have attempted to prevent speech from becoming a discriminated aversive stimulus.

In the child who is conscious of difficulty, and in whom the strength of the fear is becoming strong enough to motivate increasing deviation in the fluency pattern, the objectives—in addition to those just mentioned—are to reduce the learned or acquired fear and to extinguish the habit strength of the stuttering. Before proceeding into this more direct type of therapy, the clinician should be certain that the less direct approach of dealing with stimulus events—or as I have said, those subject and environmental variables which occasion disfluency—will not be sufficient. This involves a careful judgment. Most clinicians have adopted the policy of being less direct at first. As they come to know the child better, decisions are made concerning the advisability of more direct stuttering therapy.

For my own frame of reference as a clinician, and for the purpose of training clinicians, I have viewed stuttering therapy for those commonly classified as secondary stutterers as including four general areas of therapeutic activity:

1. Changing the perceptions, attitudes, and feelings of the stutterer.

2. Extinguishing fear and avoidance behavior related to sounds, words, and speaking situations.

3. Diminishing excessive bodily tension.

4. Building up new psychomotor speech patterns.

In thinking of stuttering therapy all four of these objectives and/or areas of activity are considered to be interrelated and, in general, are approached almost simultaneously, although one may be emphasized more during a certain period of therapy. I have found it helpful—and other speech clinicians have also reported it to be beneficial—to think of these general areas as dimensions of improvement to which attention should be given in a total approach to the problem. Perhaps the comment should be inserted that, although approaches have to be modified with every case, it has been found useful to follow a general frame of reference, and, to some extent, even a general sequence or course of activities in working with stutterers. Therefore, I shall discuss the management of stuttering and the applications of learning theory concepts with reference to these four areas. For reasons which will be stated later, I shall first consider work with secondary stutterers of approximately age ten or older and adult stutterers. Later I should like to show how these procedures are modified in working with younger secondary stutterers of the early elementary school age.

CHANGING THE STUTTER'S PERCEPTIONS, ATTITUDES, AND FEELINGS

Diverse results have characterized the research findings pertaining to the personality and adjustment of stutterers, but most commentaries on the literature, while not reporting the finding of a particular personality pattern that is characteristic of stutterers, do conclude that stutterers appear to be somewhat more anxious, tense, and withdrawn (Johnson, 1956; Goodstein, 1958). Although there is no systematic personality difference (Sheehan, 1958a), there seems to be general agreement that stutterers possess certain attitudes about speech and speaking which cause anxiety and insecurity in interpersonal relations, for example, their severe rejection of hesitant speech in general and stuttering speech in particular.

I suggest that in working with stutterers attitudes be viewed as mediating responses (Allport, 1935; Mowrer, 1960a, 1960b), these responses representing degrees of positive (associated with hope) and negative (associated with fear) expectation resulting from experiences with certain persons, groups, and situations (stimuli). In turn, these attitudinal responses can act as stimuli to varying degrees of approach or avoidance behavior (responses).[1] Therefore, a chain of events in the making of a speech response to be dealt with in stuttering therapy can be schematically illustrated in Figure 23.

If the expectation (R_a, attitudinal response) toward certain stimuli (as illustrated in the above diagram) is predominantly one of comfort and pleasure, then the response that follows would be mainly one of approach; but if it were to a greater degree one of discomfort, the response would be mainly one of avoidance; or there could be an approach-avoidance conflict.[2]

1. Based on Mowrer's revised two-factor theory of learning. See Mowrer (1960a, 1960b) and Chap. 1, this volume.
2. For a discussion of stuttering as an approach-avoidance conflict, see Sheehan (1958b) and Chap. 5, this volume.

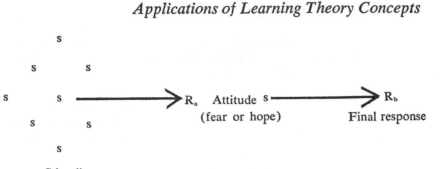

Fɪɢ. 23.—A schematic illustration of the principal events in the chain of oc-currences in a speech response which can be dealt with in stuttering therapy.

Applying this frame of reference to stuttering, it is hypothesized that certain mediating mal-attitudes or negative expectancies arise in the stutterer as he experiences noxious stimulation in the presence of certain persons or in certain situations; this noxious stimulation gradually becomes generalized to sounds and words.[3]

One common attitude which, undoubtedly, most clinicians have observed in stutterers is that all hesitant speech is abnormal. Johnson (1946, 1956) has traced the development of this sensitive attitude. He points out that the stutterer hesitates to hesitate (1946). Therefore, hesitant speech as a stimulus brings about a fear response (negative expectation), because the stutterer has adopted the attitude that hesitant speech is abnormal. Feelings or emotions, often labeled as shame or embarrassment, are analogous mediating responses; in other words, negative expectation and fear are involved. These attitudes act as stimulus cues to avoidance behavior.

Another prevalent attitude of the stutterer is one of hostility toward those who react to his stuttering in any of a variety of ways. This attitude of hostility as a response may then act as a cue for aggressive behavior. Extending this example and assuming that stimulus generalization operates in stutterers just as it does in others, the stutterer comes to make a similar response to people other than those who originally punished his speech behavior. The psychological defense mechanism of projection may operate as he perceives an attitude in others which may not actually exist but is a projection of the stutterer's own attitude.

3. Refer to Wischner (1950) for a discussion of the development of stuttering as a learned response to previously neutral cues.

In therapy, one of the ways that we go about modifying mediating attitudinal responses is by helping the stutterer to clarify and alter his thinking. I should like to mention here, but emphasize in the next section of the paper, that changes made in final responses (R_b in Fig. 23) also have an impact on our thinking and our attitudinal responses. In fact, there appears to be a reciprocal relationship between changes made in attitudinal responses and final responses. In this connection, I should like to point out that the clinician is essentially an operator in the field of language, going about this work in the following specific ways:

1. He searches out with the client certain attitudes as revealed by the client's verbal report.
2. He helps the client acquire new verbal labels, in other words, new terminology which helps him to extend his understanding of his attitudinal and overt behavioral responses.
3. He selectively rewards certain statements made by the client which he considers as indicating a change of thinking in the desired direction.
4. He makes certain interpretations which are appropriately timed.

Let me clarify these procedures by setting forth a general sequence of events through which I have found it is quite often useful to move in a therapy program.

During the early stages of both individual and group therapy sessions, a great deal of emphasis is placed upon helping the clients to feel as accepted and comfortable as possible. It is important that the therapy atmosphere have a calming effect on the stutterer as this will, by reducing anxiety and tension, enable him to verbalize attitudes more readily. In the clinician, the stutterers begin to recognize an informed person, a person with prestige, so to speak, who will listen and try to understand their feelings of frustration and humiliation. The clinician attempts to comprehend how the individual stutterer feels about his problem, what he thinks caused it, what he thinks others think about stuttering, what he has done previously to help himself, what he thinks has helped him, and the like. In this process, while the clinician is getting a better understanding of the person's difficulty, the client is initiating the process of re-evaluating and reorganizing his ideas.

To those clinicians who have had only a little experience thus far with stuttering therapy, I should like to mention that earlier in my clinical experience I seemed to have considerable need to impress clients with

112

how much I knew. When people come to a clinician for help, I think it is important that they know he can help. Usually, education and position take care of this to the extent necessary to motivate the person to communicate. I want to emphasize that I do not believe I have ever had a client leave therapy because I was making an honest attempt to understand him as a person with a problem. The clinician can offer reaction, comments, and possibly some information (more about the giving of information later), but what should be emphasized here is that this be done in such a way that the client feels the clinician is talking "with him," not "at him." It is crucial to the entire treatment process that the stutterer feel free to express his feelings and relate his experiences in this newly established relationship.

I certainly do not consider myself a nondirective therapist, but taking a cue from the work of Rogers (1951), there seems to be little doubt that as a person begins to talk, he begins to evaluate his ideas, reorganize his thinking, and behave somewhat differently. In addition, with reference to the clinical observation that punishment of stuttering behavior is generalized to the act of discussing it (i.e., stutterers are reticent to talk about their speech problem), this opportunity to talk—talk, in fact, being rewarded by the clinician—will help to extinguish the client's anxiety. Extinction is taking place because the previously punished, and therefore inhibited, verbal responses are now occurring without punishment. Counterconditioning, defined as a situation in which the consequence of behavior is shifted, is operating because the clinician actually *rewards* the client's talking about his problem and deconfirms the client's expectation of rejection (punishment).[4]

These statements about the early stage of therapy should imply the importance of a certain kind of relationship between the clinician and the client. Dr. Murray emphasized,[5] based on his research, that the effectiveness of reinforcers such as verbal statements depended upon the basic relationship between the client and clinician. I think clinicians should learn to establish relationships with all types of people. This is an important characteristic of a speech clinician and brings up many interesting questions about matching clients and clinicians. However, the approach I am suggesting is one way of helping client and clinician

4. Additional discussion of the extinction and counterconditioning processes is found later in this paper. See also Mowrer's discussion of unlearning in Chap. 1 of this volume. For a specific consideration of the extinction process as related to the fear of talking about certain topics, see Dollard and Miller (1950).

5. See Chap. 2 in this volume; see also Murray (1964).

113

establish a correct therapeutic environment in which to initiate a profitable relationship.

Continuing with the delineation of the commonly occurring events in therapy, it is usually apparent, following these initial explorations, that there is considerable disagreement and confusion among the clients about the problem of stuttering. Consequently, it has been found that stutterers welcome the opportunity to improve their understanding of the problem. In this phase, the objective is to give the stutterer the best general explanation available as to how stuttering behavior originates and develops. Thus, he will have an increased appreciation of the rational basis for therapy to follow. Recalling my earlier comment that we talk "with" and not "at" the client, the discussion approach encouraging an easy exchange of ideas must be continued as this information is given.

Speech development is traced from the first words to conversational speech, giving special attention to the concept of normal nonfluency. In exploring ways in which stuttering might develop—since no certainty about etiology exists—it has been found advisable to mention several alternatives. The stutterer is told that some speech pathologists believe it could be due to a parent's reaction to the normally disfluent speech of a child. On the other hand, parents and others may become concerned with, and react to, what some specialists in the field recognize as a qualitatively different kind of disfluency in a child's speech. An individual difference in emotional sensitivity could influence a particular child in either of these two situations. The stutterer comes to understand that his problem has to be evaluated carefully to discover the specific factors which may have contributed to the development of his stuttering—a minimal language deficit, a problem of motor patterning, and so forth. He begins to see that therapy will center on these factors, as well as the many common attitudes and behavior patterns (which can be traced rather definitively) characterizing stuttering.

As the client continues to discuss the problem with his clinician, each providing the other with information, the client acquires new verbal labels, which are then utilized in evaluating or thinking about his condition. Other members of the family—wives, mothers, fathers—may be going through this same process if, in the clinician's judgment, they should be included.[6] As the growth of stuttering behavior in a child is

6. Bringing other persons into the therapy process is discussed later in this section.

traced, such labels as "secondary mannerisms," "starters," "avoidances," and "hard contacts" are acquired and their meanings attached. Almost immediately, but in varying degrees, clients will begin to attach these meanings in differing ways to specific stimulus events and responses. Labels and new ideas may aid the person in describing a memory of some previous experience, such as being teased about his stuttering, or the way in which he developed a secondary mannerism. Later in treatment, these labels help the client to evaluate some learning experience, such as the playing of a role, which the clinician arranges in the clinic. In this connection, verbal labels have great utility in helping the person to think about behavior modifications. They act as cues to more appropriate action.[7]

One goal of this labeling procedure is to alter the person's evaluation of speech fluency. As stated previously, hesitant speech becomes a stimulus for a fear response (negative expectation) because it has been punished. The fear response acts as a cue to avoidance behavior. The stutterer needs to understand that he has overgeneralized and that most non-stutterers also show considerable hesitation. He is encouraged to make a discrimination (i.e., to see the similarities and differences) between stimulus conditions of childhood and the present. To point this out, I often say, "I'm not the one who punished your stuttering. How do you know how I am reacting to it? How do you know how other people are reacting to it?" Actually, I am implying that under the proper conditions of therapy he should stop reacting like a child and begin to re-evaluate and change his behavior. I say, "Now, you are able to evaluate your behavior and determine changes on a volitional level. This was much less possible earlier and especially when you were a child. In therapy, we are going to help by creating some special circumstances in which you can begin to practice new attitudes and new behavior."

Furthermore, he must see that his severe rejection of stuttering and hesitant speech in general has come to have the effect of a vicious circle: more fear, more avoidance behavior, more speech disintegrating tension, and so forth, resulting in more stuttering. Making the discriminations (seeing the differences) between normal disfluency and stuttering, between the stimulus conditions of childhood and the present, and then recognizing the nature of this vicious circle establishes an important part of the rationale for utilizing procedures to reduce the fear of stuttering

7. See Dollard and Miller (1950) for a further discussion of labeling, and Kimble (1961) for a consideration of the role of cues in bringing about more adaptive behavior.

and to work toward changing, rather than stopping, the stuttering behavior.

From an exploration of the development and influence of these attitudes and feelings, which are very specific to speech, the scope of the self-study portion of the program is broadened to include a consideration of the dynamics of personal adjustment. Basically, I have approached this through a study of the various defense mechanisms.[8] Again, verbal labeling is an important procedure which helps the client to discriminate, as he is able to think and talk about his general behavior in terms of such concepts as compensation, rationalization, and projection. As a part of the self-study program, with reference to his general personality structure and mode of adjustment, the stutterer needs to examine the possibility that his speech handicap has had a protective effect by helping him to rationalize many life events. Oftentimes the stuttering has been overemphasized because it was convenient to use it as a rationalization for not getting a desired job or for not making the best grades in the classroom. With reference to this secondary reward aspect of stuttering, some speech pathologists have spoken of the stutterer's strong tendency to regard it as his only liability, and to adopt the attitude that if only he could speak fluently he would be like a giant released from chains. It is readily seen that these attitudes might impede progress in therapy.

EXTINGUISHING FEAR AND AVOIDANCE BEHAVIOR RELATED TO SOUNDS, WORDS, AND SPEAKING SITUATIONS

There has been a great deal of interest in the relationship between the expectation of stuttering, the ensuing anxiety, and the resulting avoidance behavior which is said to be the stuttering (Wischner, 1950; Johnson, 1955).[9] Wischner (1950) and Sheehan (1953a) have hypothesized that the confirmation of the expected difficulty and the release from the block when stuttering occurs is accompanied by a reduction of the generated anxiety and tension, and therefore the behavior (the head jerk, eye blink, lip pressure, and the like, of the stuttering block) is reinforced. With reference to the schematic illustration of the chain of

8. The material in *Know Yourself* by B. Bryngelson, *et al.* (1950) has proved valuable in this self-study program.

9. Actually, Wischner (1950) hypothesized that stuttering behavior may represent breakdown in the speech behavior consequent to the anxiety or that the acquired anxiety motivates avoidance behavior.

116

events in a stuttering response (Fig. 23), R_b (final response) represents this avoidance behavior.

As the stutterer acquires information about stuttering and gains insight into the ways in which his attitudes perpetuate the problem, increased emphasis in therapy is placed on a study and modification of the outward manifestations of stuttering behavior and the use of "fear-dosing" techniques to diminish the anxious anticipation of stuttering and to help the person approach speaking with greater assurance and hope of success. This statement indicates again what I mentioned previously: there is a reciprocal relationship between changes made in final responses and attitudinal responses. Specific examples of this will be given as particular techniques are described.

As part of the information-giving aspect of therapy, which continues throughout the treatment process, the client should come to see how his stuttering has developed. In short, he understands our postulates, based on the best research available, that punishment of his speech behavior leads to fear (portrayed eventually as certain attitudes), which, in turn, motivates avoidance behavior (stuttering). He acquires labels for avoidance behavior such as "starter," "postponement," "word substitution," "circumlocution," and the like, which he usually begins to apply to his own speech. But now there is a more direct approach to the analysis and description (labeling) of the stuttering behavior as the client learns, in gradual steps, to listen to himself on the tape recorder and to study his speech behavior in the mirror. I want to emphasize the gradual approach here because it is painful for a person to examine his stuttering.

Proceeding under the assumption, one on which most clinicians agree, that the stutterer's anxiety will be somewhat increased at this point, he will need a great deal of support. I have found that the use of the verbal cue, "This takes courage," is very helpful. I say, "This is not easy, it takes courage." It does take courage and I think this is the proper label for it, a label for a positive attitude which in our society has usually come to have a hopeful, pleasant meaning. To most of us it means to try something difficult, try something a little dangerous and see if you can succeed. Another way to look at this is to say that the verbal cue, "courage," is a conditioned positive reinforcer (Staats and Staats, 1964).

As the stutterer analyzes what he is doing when he stutters and gains insight into his largely unconscious, reflexive speech patterns, he is taught and encouraged to imitate his stuttering behavior during the individual and group therapy sessions. As he practices stuttering blocks on purpose, he and the clinician label such aspects of behavior as "hard lip contact," "dilation of the nostrils," "jaw tremor," and so forth. The stutterer is instructed to sense carefully the tactile-kinesthetic feedback as these conditions of the stuttering block occur. Clinicians will recognize this as an application of Dunlap's negative practice procedure to stuttering therapy in a manner very much like that in which it has been utilized for over thirty years. In my own clinical practice, I have used this procedure extensively as a clinical exercise to help the stutterer to explore and gain insight into his speech behavior. I have not had the stutterer attempt this technique outside the clinic, where, in my opinion, the pressure is almost always so great that, if the stutterer comes this close to his habitual stuttering pattern, it will quite often, to use Van Riper's term, "trigger" an involuntary pattern. Wischner (1965) has suggested that, in using negative practice, the speech pathologist should take advantage of reactive inhibition [10] by having the stutterer utilize mass trials, in other words, have the individual make the same response over and over again very rapidly.

As a result of the experimentation which occurs during negative practice, the stutterer, with the assistance of the clinician, begins to realize that his speech blocks can be altered by relaxing the tension, slowing the repetition, and the like. To give an example, I might say, as the client is using negative practice, "Why, George, it seems to me that you changed that a little that time, that you did not push so hard. Let's look at that in the mirror again." Clinical observation and the statements of clients indicate that at this stage of therapy the stutterer's attitude of negative expectation and hopelessness related to fear (see R_a, Fig. 23) begins to shift toward an attitude of positive expectation and hope because he begins to see that this previously involuntary, reflexive activity can be modified. If the client verbalizes this reflection, it should be rewarded by the clinician, but if the client does not hit upon this thought, it should be stated for him.

At this point in the progression of events in therapy, additional ways to modify the speech response, labeled for the client as "voluntary

10. For a discussion of the concept of reactive inhibition and the associated concept of conditioned inhibition, see Hull (1943), Mowrer (1960a), and Wolpe (1958). In the application to negative practice in stuttering therapy, it is assumed that some amount of the reactive inhibition, or a fatigue associated state which accumulates with the repetition of the nonrewarded stuttering behavior, is conditioned to stimuli present when the response is made. Subsequently these stimuli will to some degree be conditioned to an inhibition of the response. Theoretically, this is why the response will be weakened.

stuttering," are introduced. Traditionally, in the avoidance-reduction method of stuttering therapy (Bryngelson, 1950; Johnson, 1946, 1956; Sheehan, 1953a, 1958b; Van Riper, 1963), two approaches to voluntary stuttering have been employed. One approach, known as the "bounce," involves a smooth, easy repetition of a syllable in a word, usually the first syllable, but it could be any one in the word. The second most widely used method of voluntary stuttering is the "slide," in which the person practices a smooth, easy approach to a syllable with a slight prolongation of the consonant continuant vowel combination or the vowel in the case of syllables beginning with stop consonants. Most modifications which stutterers use are combinations or variations of these two.

The voluntary stuttering pattern should be varied, but it should always be performed just as planned. It may be employed on feared words, but at least 50 per cent of the time it should be used on words about which there is no apprehension. Since the stutterer is beginning to do intentionally what he has such a strong tendency to avoid, the therapist again provides support by perhaps pointing out that this takes a great deal of courage. Moreover, of even greater significance at this time in therapy, the clinician, by rewarding the client for his voluntary stuttering, is managing the therapeutic situation so that the focus of reward is being changed from attempting to talk fluently and to hide stuttering, to being more willing to express the stuttering behavior and making it the object of study. The process involved here is counterconditioning, defined either as a change in reinforcement (for example, rewarding a response that has previously been punished), or as extinction (which is hastened by the reinforcement of a response displacing the original conditioned response). Summarizing this point, rewarding disfluency is changing the reinforcement, and rewarding a controlled modification (new response) is hastening the decrement of the involuntary stuttering behavior. In addition, these final behavioral response changes (R_b in Fig. 23) have an impact on the attitudinal response. The attitudinal mediating response is changing in the direction of a greater degree of positive expectation and a feeling of hope when certain stimulus complexes are present which formerly meant a greater degree of negative expectation, feeling of discomfort, and desire to avoid.

In order for these changes or modifications in the overt behavioral responses to produce the maximum effect on attitude, it is important that the purpose of the procedures be clearly labeled and understood. Therefore, when the stutterer does voluntary stuttering, he says to himself, "I am doing the thing I fear. Also, I realize that I can change my speech; I can tell my speech mechanism what to do." In this way it seems that he is able to reward himself. In contrast, some stutterers report, when asked why they were using voluntary stuttering, "That was just the thing I was told to do. Whenever I was afraid I was going to stutter, I would bounce."

As the stutterer continues to work on voluntary stuttering, he may be introduced to another fear-dosing procedure known as "cancellation" (Van Riper, 1954, 1963). This consists of learning to stop after a stuttered word and then to say it again with less struggle or using some type of voluntary stuttering. The cancellation is not successful until the word is produced under voluntary control. Beyond the opportunity to continue to study the speech pattern through a contrast of the involuntary block and the voluntary cancellation, it is hypothesized that this technique diminishes the reinforcement of the stuttering act, which, as mentioned earlier, Wischner (1950) and Sheehan (1953a) have postulated occurs when the person filibusters through a speech block and allows the behavior to be reinforced because anxiety was reduced at the immediate point in time of the occurrence of the stuttering. However, when cancellation is done, the competing, altered response is reinforced also. Speaking from my own practical experience, I have found cancellation to be a rather difficult technique for stutterers to use. Thus, when the stutterer cancels 50 per cent to 70 per cent of his blocks in the clinic, this is judged to be proficient.

Van Riper (1963), the originator of the cancellation technique, suggests that the stutterer go on to "pull-outs" after he learns to cancel. Pull-outs consist of the person not allowing the speech block to run its course, but modifying the behavior as the word is spoken. Again, the reinforcement of the maladaptive stuttering response is diminished and the adaptive pull-out is reinforced. The last step in this sequence is the preparatory set in which the adaptive, altered behavior moves forward in time, and the person is able to use his experience to approach the word more appropriately in terms of a normal speech response.

Other types of behavior, such as "delayed response," and the like, are examples of response modifications. In all of these instances, counterconditioning is being employed on the overt, final response level. When certain stimuli are present, a modified response is reinforced.

I hasten to emphasize that, in terms of the approach-avoidance concept of conflict, the clinician is motivating the person to attempt these new responses after having considerably reduced anxiety by working

120

with mediating responses, that is to say, after changing attitudes, feelings, and perceptions.[11] Moreover, it is therapeutically important to use a gradual desensitization approach in which responses are changed, first in the presence of stimuli which evoke minimal anxiety, and then in stimulus situations that have a history of producing more anxiety. One of the major contributions of therapy is that the clinician arranges a graded series of relearning situations for the client and provides guidance and encouragement as the client generalizes new responses to varying stimulus complexes. Responses become surer and more precise as practice continues. In summary, both stimulus conditions and responses have to be manipulated in the therapeutic process.

Working with my students in training and discussing the use of these fear-dosing modification procedures with practicing clinicians, I have come to believe that there is a need to be more thorough and systematic in teaching these various techniques. In my classes I point out that there is a similarity, often not recognized, between articulation therapy, voice therapy, and stuttering therapy in that these speech response changes need to be taught beginning with word lists, then proceeding to sentences and gradually to conversational speech emphasizing one speech sound at a time, for example, "b." In other words, I am very specific in teaching the stutterer how to stutter voluntarily on various sounds, vowels, consonant and vowel combinations, and so forth. (This also applies to the teaching of other fear-dosing speech modifications such as cancellations, pull-outs, and preparatory sets.) Stutterers with whom I have worked have a tendency, when employing a "bounce" pattern, to say "du-du-du-day," rather than "da-da-da-day." The former, in my opinion, is much less effective than the latter, and, indeed, is incorrect. The person should get the feeling of the smooth transition in the consonant-vowel combination together with the feeling that at any moment he wishes he can go ahead and say the word; therefore, the proper first syllable should be practiced. I have found this approach to be very effective in helping the person gain a greater sense of security with reference to his ability to perform the modification. In addition to this system of beginning with simplified material and smaller units and working up to more complex material, various techniques, such as volun-

11. Dollard and Miller (1950) and Sheehan (1953a, 1958b) have pointed out the importance of reducing avoidance before increasing approach tendencies. When there are extremely strong avoidance tendencies, increasing motivation to approach will vastly increase the fear and resulting conflict. After fear or avoidance behavior is considerably reduced, then increasing approach tendencies is more likely to produce a good effect.

tary stuttering, are used first in situations that evoke very little anxiety, and then are gradually introduced into situations of increasing stress.

DIMINISHING EXCESSIVE BODILY TENSION

It is obvious that the struggling speech behavior of the stutterer involves muscular tension. This tension appears to be an element in the vicious circle of stuttering. The stutterer responds to certain stimuli with negative expectations and fear, which, in turn, stimulate avoidance behavior involving increased tension; he then speaks less fluently and has greater negative expectation, thus setting the entire process into motion once again.

I have found that instruction in progressive and differential muscle relaxation is valuable in helping the stutterer to reduce tension during speech. Also, the stutterer's thinking of, and striving for, relaxation when under stress seems to have the effect of bringing about a general reduction of his anxiety. With reference to the latter benefit of deep muscle relaxation, Wolpe (1958) has recently emphasized its use in psychotherapy because "deep muscle relaxation has autonomic effects antagonistic to those of anxiety" (p. 135). Wolpe hypothesized that anxiety is defined by the activity of the sympathetic branch of the autonomic nervous system which results in increased palmar sweating, increased heart rate, and increased pulse rate. On the other hand, relaxation, as a response, is associated with activity of the parasympathetic branch of the autonomic nervous system which acts to inhibit the sympathetic branch. Therefore, relaxation is viewed as a response antagonistic to anxiety which, according to Wolpe, reciprocally inhibits anxiety. This phenomenon appears to be similar to counterconditioning, which is brought about by extinction under conditions where the decrement of the original response (anxiety in this case) is hastened by the reinforcement of a second response that displaces the original one.

Relaxation has sometimes been described as a method in and of itself for the treatment of stuttering. I do not believe, however, that relaxation procedures have much permanent value unless they are part of a more inclusive therapeutic process.

I have used the techniques of progressive and differential relaxation which have been described by Jacobson (1938). Briefly, the approach involves a systematic tensing and relaxing of the muscles in one part of the body at a time, beginning at the feet and working upward to the head

122

and neck. Emphasis is placed on developing a sensory awareness of the intermediate gradations of muscle tone. The conditioning of verbal cues to be associated with the motor activity is brought about as the clinician, at first, tells the client to feel carefully the increase in tension in, for example, the arm, and then tells him to focus on the change as the tension decreases. Finally, the client is told to "talk to himself" (give himself instructions) as he voluntarily tenses and relaxes specific muscle groups. The client is given the following rationale for the relaxation procedure:

1. In order to relieve the tension of the speech mechanism, one must learn to be aware of the state of tension in the small and large muscle groups throughout the body.
2. Thinking of and striving for increased relaxation when under stress will provide a competing response which will help one to be calmer.

For purposes of clearer exposition, I have discussed the use of relaxation at this point, but in practice these exercises are begun very early in therapy. The learning which takes place, related to this particular area of activity, is integrated with work in other areas as therapy progresses.

BUILDING UP NEW PSYCHOMOTOR SPEECH PATTERNS

If speech is considered as a psychomotor response (a motor response which occurs under varying or changing psychological circumstances), then as maladaptive speech responses are weakened through the use of fear-dosing speech modifications (described previously), new speech responses—or psychomotor speech patterns—must be practiced and strengthened. Actually, this process begins as the stutterer learns to modify his speech by using negative practice, voluntary stuttering, cancellation, pull-out, preparatory set, delayed response, and so forth, but in this section I am emphasizing the practice, by the stutterer, of certain speech behavior (R_b in Fig. 23), which he has most likely never acquired because talking has often been for him such a fearful, frustrating experience.

Recently, Goldiamond (1965) has used delayed auditory feedback in establishing and shaping a new speech pattern. A prolonged speech pattern, which is under the control of novel stimuli (delayed auditory feedback), is brought under the control of more general stimuli by decreasing the delay of the auditory feedback as the shaping of the

123

response occurs. This technique appears to be appropriate in terms of the objective being discussed here.

In using the delayed auditory feedback procedure, a tape recorder which provides one delay time may be used and the loudness of the delayed signal decreased systematically (Gross and Gregory, 1966; Gross and Nathanson, 1967), or a recorder-playback system may be used in which the delay can be adjusted (Goldiamond, 1965). In brief, the procedure, as we have employed it, is to instruct the subject, beginning with reading, to use a slow, prolonged pattern of speech which enables him to overcome the negative or punishing effects of the delayed feedback. The delay can be faded out gradually in the use of a system with a variable delay control. In a system with a fixed delay, the loudness can be decreased gradually; then the delay can be eliminated. A similar program is then carried out in spontaneous speech, beginning with less propositional responses, such as answers to routine questions, and moving in gradual steps to more meaningful communication. Finally, the subject is instructed to instate the pattern volitionally without delayed auditory feedback, beginning, as before, with less propositional speech. The rate and pattern can be modified in gradual steps.[12]

At that time in therapy when avoidance tendencies are diminishing and approach tendencies are increasing, improvement of speech skills is stressed by teaching appropriate rate control (through the use of phrasing and the proper duration of vowel sounds), better vocal inflection, and an increased awareness of the variations in articulatory force which can be used in producing sounds. The stutterer's speech behavior is "shaped" as the clinician suggests or demonstrates these skills and rewards the client as he approximates the new behavior. The significance of this activity is that it increases even further the stutterer's positive expectations, feelings of hope, and approach tendencies, as contrasted to his negative expectations and avoidance tendencies. At the same time, the new final speech responses are generalized more extensively to other stimuli as the stutterer practices in situations of real life.

12. There is presently considerable discussion of the utilization of this procedure in stuttering therapy. My present opinion is that this technique is beneficial when used as part of a complete approach as outlined in this chapter. Future study may reveal advantages of its use with subjects of a certain age, or as progress is made in differential evaluation, we may be able to determine the specific clients with whom it is desirable to use this or one of the similar approaches to initiating a new psychomotor speech pattern. In addition, we need to study the advantages and disadvantages of using this approach earlier in the therapeutic process than has been indicated in this discussion.

THE FACILITATION OF CHANGE OUTSIDE THE CLINIC

Traditionally, in speech therapy, clinicians have accompanied stutterers on "field trips" and given them assignments of practicing new behavior in "nucleus" situations outside the clinic. Clinicians have always emphasized that altered thinking and behavior in the clinic must be accompanied by a change of behavior in relevant life situations.

To facilitate this generalization, or transfer, of altered attitudes, speech responses, and social responses to persons and situations outside the clinic, I have utilized an "open clinic," group therapy approach in which the stutterer's family, his friends, and other interested persons are encouraged to participate in the discussions and activities of the group sessions. Everyone—client, clinician, and visitors—is encouraged to say whatever he likes. Valuable group catharsis (anxiety extinction) takes place as the stutterers and non-stutterers share experiences; and self-centeredness, appearing in stutterers in the form of overconcern about the problem, diminishes as the stutterers listen to the non-stutterers discuss their problems. Furthermore, significant persons in the everyday life of the client have the opportunity to see how the therapist is teaching new responses and shifting reinforcements. Thus, those individuals who associate with the client are able to support the clinician's therapeutic effort. Finally, this approach provides an appropriate setting for the use of role-playing techniques in which the stutterer practices new behavior patterns in more of a real life situation.

To determine the situations which will be worked on during the role playing, the stutterer is asked to list speaking situations in a descending order of difficulty. The clinician then leads the group in planning carefully graded relearning experiences, beginning with the least difficult situations. After role playing a situation one to several times during the group sessions, the stutterer is assigned to work on the situation in real life.

Miller (1964) has urged psychotherapists to examine more extensively the use of this kind of social group or community approach in terms of its value in extinction, counterconditioning, and generalization.

THERAPY FOR THE YOUNG SECONDARY STUTTERER

Over the years, I have experienced especial difficulty in working with moderately severe to severe secondary stutterers between the ages of six or seven and ten or eleven. The general objectives—spelled out in the

125

four areas of therapeutic activity and the basic principles of learning which I have already discussed—appear applicable; however, as has been generally recognized by clinicians, certain modifications in approach have to be made in consideration of the child's social maturity and level of intellectual development.

Piaget's description of the child (see Flavell, 1963), aged seven to eleven, as passing through the period of "concrete operations" is important in determining the extent to which we can utilize intellectualized therapy approaches, such as those discussed in this chapter, in changing the attitudes, perceptions, and feelings of the child. According to Piaget, the child from seven to eleven deals most effectively with the reality before him; whereas, in the period of "formal operations," ages eleven to fifteen, the child can also deal with the world of pure possibility, the world of abstract, propositional statements, the world of "as-if."

During the last eight years, I have developed and taught my students the system described below for working with the speech behavior of the young secondary stutterer. This system—which emphasizes activities in the two areas of extinguishing fear and avoidance behavior and building up new psychomotor speech patterns—appears to offer several advantages, including that of creating in the child a feeling of security which comes from dealing with concrete procedures which are repeated routinely and often. In addition, the units of stuttered speech can be controlled, making it more possible for the child and clinician to examine some segment of the child's stuttering behavior under conditions in which the ratio of stuttering to fluent speech is decreased. Also, the child approaches the analysis of his own speech gradually, and, very importantly, always after studying "stuttering" in the clinician's speech. The threat of examining this behavior, which he dreads and tries to avoid, is thus greatly diminished. The emphasis upon looking at this behavior first in the clinician's speech, even though it is initiated voluntarily by the clinician, seems to be reinforcing to the child, since an example is being set by what learning theorists would call a "reinforcing agent."

The system may be outlined as follows:

Step 1. Tape record client and clinician reading chorally. Read at child's pace. Begin with word lists, proceed to phrases, sentences, and paragraph material. Play back.

Step 2. Same as Step 1, but with microphone nearer the child. Play back. Child hears his relatively fluent speech in the foreground of the recording.

126

Step 3. Tape record choral reading. Microphone nearer clinician. Clinician has one to several stuttering blocks. Play back. Child and clinician listen to clinician's blocks. They look at the clinician's "stoppages" in the mirror. The clinician and child describe what is happening to the clinician's speech.

Each step is always begun with words and works up to longer units. At the first one or two sessions, Steps 1 and 2 only may be used. Step 3 may be reached during the third or fourth session. *Every* session always begins with Step 1 and works up to an appropriate point in the system.

Step 4. Choral reading again. Clinician drops out and allows child to have one to several blocks and then picks up choral reading again. Thus, the clinician is usually able to control the extent of the child's stuttering behavior. On playbacks, child and clinician listen and later look at the child's stuttering behavior. Just previous to this, they have, as was done on every occasion before, looked and listened first to the clinician's speech, in which he has initiated stuttering blocks of various types.

Step 5. Same as Step 4, adding negative practice in which the child voluntarily imitates his stuttering blocks.

Step 6. Choral reading (always using a tape recorder) in which the child is taught voluntary stuttering (example: bounce and slide patterns), and it is emphasized that he can tell his speech mechanism what to do; also, that he is doing on purpose what he has been afraid to do and has tried to avoid. Here, hopefully, attitudes are being changed within the child's specific experience. It has been found important to teach these modifications precisely and carefully, using word lists representing various consonant sounds. As previously, work up to sentences, paragraph material, short answers to questions, and finally conversation.

Step 7. More and more emphasis on new psychomotor responses, emphasizing light contacts, smooth transitions, phrasing, loudness and pitch variation, and so forth.

In every session, the clinician begins with Step 1 and works up to the appropriate point in the system. During a session, the sequence of steps being employed may be repeated several times. As therapy proceeds, steps may be abbreviated or omitted, depending on the child's response.

127

Work on relaxation procedures and other therapeutic activities appropriate for an individual child can be integrated with this approach to diminishing the fear and avoidance behavior and to building up a new psychomotor speech response. As indicated previously, the system outlined above is deemed important with particular regard to the child's developing conceptual abilities. Therefore, therapy directed specifically toward a restructuring of the child's thinking about his problem, his verbal formulas—the mediating attitudes—has to be appropriate to the child's daily experience. I find it especially crucial to explain a concept concretely by giving examples which make specific reference to a child in a life situation similar to that of the child in therapy.

SUMMARY

Stuttering therapy, viewed as an application of learning theory concepts of extinction, counterconditioning, generalization, and discrimination, has been described in terms of specific techniques in four general areas of therapeutic activity:
1. Changing perceptions, attitudes, and feelings of stutterers;
2. Extinguishing fear and avoidance behavior;
3. Diminishing excessive bodily tension;
4. Building up new psychomotor speech patterns.

A schematic diagram (see Fig. 23) of the principal events (various stimuli, attitudinal responses, and final responses) in the chain of occurrences in a speech response which can be dealt with in stuttering therapy was discussed as an additional frame of reference for illustrating the relationship between therapeutic procedures in these four main areas. Learning and/or relearning in the case of the young secondary stutterer was considered with special regard to the child's level of conceptual development. Reference was also made to the importance of evaluating certain individual differences, some of which could be due to a maturational lag or an organic deficit, that should be considered in stuttering therapy.

VIII

HUGO H. GREGORY

Summary, Conclusions, Implications

THE PAPERS PRESENTED IN THIS BOOK are ample evidence that learning theory occupies a place of considerable importance in the continuing attempt to improve our understanding of the onset, development, and maintenance of stuttering, and, furthermore, that present-day stuttering therapies are based largely on psychological learning principles. It may be useful in this last chapter to summarize concisely some of the main points that have been made, making reference to areas of agreement and disagreement, indicating possible conclusions, and looking at implications for the future. Another purpose of these concluding remarks will be to describe briefly, and to offer comment upon, some work which is of considerable significance but which was not covered specifically in the symposium papers.

MOWRER, DOLLARD AND MILLER, AND SKINNER

Mowrer's review of the historical developments in the psychology of learning, which led to his own contributions, included a comparison of Pavlov's interest in stimulus-substitution learning (classical conditioning) and Thorndike's view that learning was a matter of changing the response (trial-and-error learning, instrumental learning). He also comments briefly on the work of Tolman and Hull.

In the revised two-factor theory of learning, instead of attempting to explain some learning as Pavlovian and some learning as Thorndikian, all learning is seen as involving classical conditioning or sign learning. External stimuli or response-produced stimuli come to be "signs" of fear or hope (secondary reinforcement) and thus bring about avoidance behavior and/or inhibition of behavior (associated with fear) or approach behavior and/or facilitation of behavior (associated with hope). According to Mowrer, this theory is still "two-factored," in the sense that learning occurs under two different conditions of reinforcement, drive reduction (reward) and drive induction (punishment).

Mowrer also states that our understanding of secondary reinforcement is enhanced considerably by this way of viewing behavior. This is important, as we are coming to see more and more the significance of secondary reinforcement in the development of behavior and in the relearning process. In addition, those who are interested in the vicarious learning which language makes possible and the manner in which language can serve as a cue for behavior will find the discussion in Mowrer (1960b) enlightening and provocative.

Murray reviews Dollard and Miller's interpretation of learning and psychotherapy beginning with a brief description of the four fundamental factors in learning: (1) drives (strong stimuli that impel responses), (2) cues (stimuli distinctive in kind and strength that guide responses), (3) responses, and (4) reinforcements (reductions of drive stimuli). Drive as strong external or internal stimulation acting on the person and the reinforcement of responses that reduce this drive are central in Dollard and Miller's theory. Murray also reviews the concepts of fear as a learned drive and approach-avoidance conflicts. Miller's contributions (1944) in these two areas are significant parts of the frame of reference used by Dollard and Miller to describe neurosis. Sheehan (1953a, 1958b) has employed the Dollard-Miller approach-avoidance conflict model to describe certain aspects of the development of stuttering, to

130

delineate the nature of the ongoing stuttering process, and to generate research hypotheses.

Wischner's (1950) hypothesis about the effects of punishment on disfluent speech and his descriptions of the way in which maladaptive reinforcement takes place in stuttering is based, to a considerable degree, on Mowrer's work pertaining to anxiety-reduction as a reinforcer.[1] As we have seen, Mowrer's revised two-factor theory encompasses the situation in which, through punishment, fear becomes attached to formerly neutral external or response-produced stimuli (e.g., speech) and, in turn, the fear motivates behavior (secondary manifestations of stuttering) which, if successful in reducing the fear, is reinforced.

Sheehan's approach-avoidance conflict theory of stuttering (Sheehan, 1953a, 1958b), although based more directly on Dollard and Miller's concepts, can probably be subsumed in Mowrer's theory. Mowrer suggests that his treatment of conflict needs to be carefully checked against Miller's studies (1944) of approach-avoidance behavior; however, he apparently thinks that the revised two-factor theory clarifies a situation of conflict, for example, where both positive, hope-producing and negative, fear-producing stimuli are present at the same time.

Most of the papers in the symposium made reference to Mowrer's theorizing and research and, as indicated above, reference is also made to the contributions of Miller and Dollard. In addition, the references to operant conditioning procedures for observing and modifying behavior which occur throughout this volume indicate that attention should be given in this summary to a concise review of the principles of operant analysis and a brief comparison of Skinner's work with that of Dollard and Miller, and with that of Mowrer.

Skinner identifies two kinds of learning, respondent conditioning and operant conditioning. Respondent conditioning, which follows the pattern of classical conditioning, pertains to the learning of responses that are elicited by a stimulus in a reflexive manner. Salivation, pupillary response to light, and the patellar reflex are examples. One eliciting stimulus can be substituted for another by classical conditioning. Skinner, however, has been more interested in operant conditioning, which follows the pattern of Thorndike's early work on instrumental behavior and pertains to the reinforcement of behavior emitted by the organism rather than that elicited by stimuli. Operant conditioning may be diagramed as follows:

1. See editor's note, pp. 6–7.

$$R\text{------}Rf \text{ stimulus.}$$

R is the response and Rf stimulus is the stimulus that is contingent upon the response and serves to reinforce it. A stimulus that is present when a response is emitted and reinforced can come to be a discriminated stimulus (S_D; see diagram below) for the response; thereby the response is brought under the control of the stimulus:

$$S_D\text{------}R\text{------}Rf \text{ stimulus.}$$

When the reinforcement is, generally speaking, rewarding to the organism (a positive reinforcer), the frequency or probability of a response is increased. On the other hand, when an emitted response is followed by a stimulus that is aversive or punishing (a negative reinforcer), the frequency or probability of the response is decreased. Skinner refers to the situation in which a response results in the removal of a punishing stimulus as negative reinforcement. Electric shock is an example of a negative reinforcer because its termination is reinforcing. Finally, when a positive reinforcer no longer follows a response, the rate of response decreases. This is extinction.

Mowrer would not dispute the behavioral changes indicated under the response contingencies just reviewed; however, he would invoke the two-factor theory to explain *why* these changes in response rate occur. For example, presentation of a positive reinforcer increases response rate because the stimuli, external and response-produced, occurring at the time of the positive reinforcement are associated with hope (a satisfying autonomic response).

Dollard and Miller, as their theory is reviewed by Murray, would interpret these changes in response rate in terms of drive reduction. For example, the presentation of a positive reinforcer increases the rate of response because the drive or need is being reduced by that reinforcing stimulus. The withdrawal of a positive reinforcer reduces response rate because the response is no longer reinforcing; in other words, it is no longer reducing drive (strong stimulation).[2]

Classical conditioning and operant conditioning come together at the

2. Two publications by Miller are expansions of his theory (which has been reviewed in this volume by Murray and has been applied to stuttering by Sheehan). Implications of current concepts of learning for behavior change are discussed in Miller (1964). Miller (1963) postulates a "go mechanism" in the brain which acts to intensify ongoing responses. He has shown greater interest in the interaction of certain neurophysiological mechanisms in learning and has referred to the involvement of the reticular activating system in the "go mechanism." The reader will be interested in Miller's reactions to Mowrer's revised two-factor theory explanation of the acquisition of skilled behavior, and so forth.

point where secondary or conditioned reinforcers are considered. Stimuli associated with a primary positive or a primary negative reinforcer can become "substitute" stimuli for the positive or negative reinforcer through a process which is essentially classical conditioning.

Skinner and his students have had a major interest in techniques for modifying responses, and without doubt one of their most significant contributions has been the study of reinforcement schedules—the quantitative relationship between reinforcer and response. Reinforcement schedules are designated as ratio and interval depending on whether the reinforcing stimulus is given following a certain number of responses or after a certain interval of time. The ratio schedule or the interval schedule can be fixed or variable. Research data has indicated the following about schedules of reinforcement:

1. The learning of a new response proceeds most rapidly when every response is reinforced. However, extinction is also most rapid when this schedule is employed.

2. After a response is acquired, a variable ratio schedule (known also as an intermittent or partial schedule) of reinforcement is best for maintaining the response rate. Utilization of this schedule also insures greater resistance to extinction.

3. Likewise, a variable ratio schedule of punishment is most effective.[3]

A lively time can usually be had by initiating a discussion on the topic of Skinner's attitude toward theory. He states explicitly that the best way to understand the development of behavior and the technology of behavior change is to restrict oneself to observables. The analysis-of-behavior approach, advocated by Skinner and the operant school, emphasizes observing emitted behavior (responses), the consequence of the behavior (the reinforcement), and the discriminating stimuli associated with the responses. What cannot be observed, what is going on inside the body, the nonemitted, nonoperant behavior, cannot be dealt with; thus, theorizing about it is of little practical value.

Mowrer, on the other hand, refers to his system as "the revised two-factor *theory* of learning." As compared to Skinner, one recognizes the importance he gives to classical conditioning; but furthermore,

---

3. Principles of operant conditioning, including the effects of scheduling of reinforcement, are discussed in detail in Ferster and Skinner (1957) and in Skinner (1959).

Mowrer is willing to talk about such emotions as fear and hope, which are certainly not readily observable (although many researchers, including Mowrer and Murray in this volume, have made reference to the operational definition of fear as it is indexed by the psychogalvanic skin response). In his paper, Mowrer speculates that stuttering may be a manifestation of realistic "guilt," in keeping with his present conception of psychopathology (1964, 1965b).[4] Mowrer is here referring to an intervening variable, a feeling which can be described verbally by a person, but which cannot be otherwise "observed." Likewise, Dollard and Miller refer to unobservables such as drive and response-produced stimuli. Miller's recent writing is highly theoretical (see n. 2, p. 132).

Dollard and Miller have emphasized the deficit in the use of the higher mental processes in neurosis and have described in detail how the clinician helps the patient to label his behavior, for example, to learn to think about it. Mowrer, in his work with people who are having difficulty in social relations, is very interested in the way in which language mediates learning. He has pointed (1965a) to the developing trend of investigators who proceed along Skinnerian lines to become interested in self-direction and self-control as effected through verbal behavior. Thus, Krasner (1958) has reported on the shaping of the verbal behavior of the patient by contingencies supplied by the therapist, and Goldiamond (1965) has spoken of the patient meeting with the therapist to learn how to analyze his behavior, profit from the knowledge of the therapist, and plan new behavior. The verbal behaviors of both therapist and patient play prominent roles in this procedure. In the paper by Goldiamond we read:

Another procedure involves self-control. This consists in training S to recognize those behaviors of his which he wants to modify. Rather than telling him to modify them (something which he may have already told himself) he is trained in the experimental analysis of behavior, and also in the variables which maintain it, or which he may recruit to modify it. The weekly therapy sessions then become research conferences, as though between a professor and his research associate on what has to be done to bring the organism's behavior into line. The S is the acknowledged expert in the content of the field—his behavior and its ecology, and E brings to bear on the problem his knowledge of procedures and past effects. Eventually, as in a good professional relation, S may become an independent investigator, capable of tending to things on his own. (pp. 153–54)

4. See also Jourard (1964).

134

Many speech clinicians have employed similar procedures of analysis and treatment in working with stutterers. I think, however, that the emphasis on this careful analysis of the behavior and the planning of action to be taken is likely to contribute to more efficient and effective therapy. Also, the strong kinship between this system and the procedures and techniques of speech clinicians is seen in the emphasis on the change of behavior and the point of view that this has an important impact upon emotions and attitudes.

Mowrer describes all unlearning and relearning as involving extinction and counterconditioning. Furthermore, he surmises that, in the final analysis, extinction and counterconditioning may be identical processes.[5] Recently, Mowrer (1965a) acknowledged that operant conditioning procedures, although "limited in their human application," may have some legitimate use. He seems to think that the emphasis on altering behavior deficits and inappropriate behavior is of particular value. Moreover, this is the main thrust of Mowrer's Integrity Therapy, in which realistic guilt feelings are counterconditioned as the person identifies his "deviant and duplicious" behavior, confesses to significant others, and finally takes responsibility to change.

In conclusion, psychotherapy based on the theories of Dollard and Miller, Mowrer, or Skinner emphasizes working with verbal behavior as well as the more overt responses of the patient. Dollard and Miller refer to the labeling of emotional reactions and the restoration of thinking. Mowrer speaks of encouraging and restoring verbal self-examination. Skinner's followers direct attention to the development of more correct verbal self-instruction and control. Dollard and Miller and Mowrer have shared a history of interest extending over several decades in the counterconditioning of emotions and in work with complex personality problems. Although interested originally in less complicated human learning, Skinner has applied operant analysis and control to psychotherapy during recent years. Skinner stresses an analysis of stimulus control (stimuli that lead to certain behaviors) and the manipulation of reinforcing stimuli in the unlearning of inappropriate behavior and the acquisition of new behavior. He is not concerned with interpretations such as drive reduction, signs attached to external and response-produced cues, or the like. Skinner accepts what he observes—that rewards are reinforcing—and goes on from there. The emphasis is on the rewarding of

5. See p. 16, this volume.

positive tendencies and on the teaching of new behavior. Dollard and Miller stress the extinction of the learned fear drive and the restoration of cue-producing responses, largely verbal labels, in the therapeutic process. As the person begins to think about his behavior, he tries new responses which are in harmony with the standards of our society and which can be rewarded. Mowrer proposes that the behavior change required in psychotherapy, and perhaps in stuttering therapy, is a verbal disclosure of realistic guilt feelings, and a personal decision to change the conduct which is producing the guilt.

The principle of counterconditioning can be used to interpret all of these approaches. The differences seem to revolve more around *what* aspect of the person's behavior should be changed. Finally, it may be that a particular interpretation results in a more fruitful approach to a certain type of desired behavior change. This has been indicated in the literature. With this in mind, we are in for an exciting time in the field of speech pathology as we continue to investigate the way in which these theories apply to the development and therapy of stuttering and other speech problems.

THE ORIGIN OF STUTTERING

Aberrant patterns of speech behavior probably enter the developmental picture of stuttering very early. However, Gregory and Luper reported clinical experience indicating that certain children may have more fluency disruptions—and possibly of a qualitatively different nature from the usual—which are associated with minimal language deficits and problems of motor speech patterning. Many cases of stuttering may involve social learning only (social learning being defined as behavior influenced by the environment), but in those cases where there is a basic deficit which may be organic, it should be revealed by careful testing and taken into consideration in therapy. Mention should also be made of my present interest in the hypothesis that the higher incidence of stuttering which is being reported in the urban, culturally deprived population is related to a lack of language learning opportunities. There is a need to know more about the development of stuttering in these children, including the age of onset.

Finally, this relates to the idea of different types of stutterers. Sheehan refers to an interest in different psychological types of stutterers. Research investigations of the relationship between problems of language at the onset of stuttering and the differential evaluation of stutterers is

136

proceeding presently in several research centers in the United States. The way in which different kinds of fluency disruption might be related to differing contributing factors or etiologies is another area which needs to be studied.

THE BEHAVIOR MODEL

As Murray has stated, behavior therapists view psychopathology as learned in the social context; therefore, they approach maladaptive behavior through a psychological, educational, or behavioral model rather than a medical model. Behavior modification involves the acquisition and changing of responses rather than the treatment of a physical or medical disease that has caused a problem. Freudian psychological theory, according to the behavior theorist and therapist, regards maladaptive behavior as the outward manifestation of unconscious causes (the medical model), whereas behavior theory emphasizes that we are dealing with learned maladaptive behavior. There is no neurosis. There is only the behavior itself.

As is often the case, the danger of being unsemantic, "either-orish," applies to this differentiation. However, all of the papers herein have implied essential agreement with the behavioral model and have emphasized that helping the person to change his behavior, and/or counseling those in the environment to modify their behavior, is the vital approach in our therapy. Some may see an element of conflict between this general principle and the main point made in the preceding section—that, in some cases, certain subject variables such as a language deficit or a motor problem, which could be due to a maturational lag or an organic deficit, may be an important contributing factor in a particular stuttering problem. Speech clinicians as a group have certainly been behavior therapists. For many years they have placed great emphasis on the benefit of direct behavior change. Clinicians have realized the need not only to modify behavior, but to make up for behavioral deficits. This has been true regardless of the source of the deficit: maturational, organic, or learned, or, as is so often the situation, a combination of these.

Finally, there are those of us who do not believe that adhering to a behavioral model precludes an interest in the physiological. Mowrer and Murray have referred to the measurement of the galvanic skin response as a verification of anxiety. Observable responses such as this can be useful in understanding the effect of certain stimulus conditions and in

137

recording other correlates of behavior changes. A related example of interest in the physiological characteristics of an individual is the interest in Europe in the neurovegetative functioning of stutterers (Arnold and Luchsinger, 1965) and the references by Beech, Eysenck, Meyer, and Walton (Eysenck, 1960) to the psychotherapeutic theory, for which they offer some verification, that "the same symptom may require different techniques of treatment, depending on the autonomic reactivity and the condition-ability of a patient" (p. 465).

THE COMPLEXITY OF STUTTERING

It has always been of great concern to those of us engaged in the modification of human behavior, whether speech clinician, psychotherapist, or teacher, that we oversimplify the behavior involved when we analyze it by referring to certain general events as stimuli and other events, for example, a stuttering block, as a response. Luper stresses this concern in his paper (see Chap. 6), and from his practical experience as a clinician he has provided an explicit example and discussion of this point. It will be recalled that he referred to the following characteristics of stuttering as ones which required further attempts at explanation through the process of theorizing, clinical observation, and research: (1) the intersubject variability of stuttering, (2) the differences usually found between stuttering in children and adults, (3) the intermittency of the occurrence of stuttering behavior, and (4) the sequential nature of the behaviors involved as contrasted to the way in which they are usually described in discrete units. Of course, one may be tempted to dismiss these issues by stating that these characteristics would be expected of a behavior that is learned. Luper, however, advises a more thorough examination of stuttering behavior with reference to sequential learning as discussed by Osgood (1953) and others.

Sequencing or motor chaining and the related concepts of response-correlated stimuli and feedback are useful in attempts to trace more definitively the development of stuttering behavior as it increases in complexity. There remains, as mentioned earlier, a need for additional longitudinal studies of the development of stuttering [6] and the way in which types of symptoms may be related to a certain etiology or etiologies of stuttering. Furthermore, it will be advantageous to improve our

6. This may be considered almost impossible. Perhaps many clinicians could learn a great deal, however, by watching what happens to their own cases that continue to become more severe.

138

ability to analyze the "links" in the stuttering chain and to work with these smaller units in therapy.

Luper also amplifies the way in which the punishing consequences administered by the environment or resulting from the difficulty of speaking, stimulus generalization, and stimulus discrimination enter into the development of stuttering. He refers to the significant theoretical paper by Shames and Sherrick (1963) when he points to the relatively stable, yet variable, nature of stuttering as possibly resulting from its being reinforced on a highly irregular schedule. As I have indicated previously, operant conditioning procedures have provided a fresh, exciting, and practical approach to the analysis of behavior and speech pathology. Shames and Sherrick describe the way in which stuttering may be "maintained by positive and negative reinforcements on complex, multiple schedules" (1963, p. 17). I also find provocative the discussion by these authors of "respondent-operant overlap" conditioning. They point out that certain autonomic responses accompany operant behavior, especially where punishment is involved. Mowrer would no doubt state that certain autonomic responses also accompany operant behavior where positive reinforcement is involved. The relationship between operant and classical conditioning and the physiological concomitants should be investigated further.

THEORY AND PRACTICE: THE THEORETICIAN AND THE CLINICIAN

In the chapter by Williams, many important warnings are sounded about problems which exist as a result of the difference in responsibilities, immediate objectives, and manner of language and thought between the theoretician and the clinician. The clinician has to make decisions with the evidence available. The theoretician has to adopt the attitude and the method of the basic scientist and delay a decision until valid and reliable data have been gathered in a systematic manner. Thus, there is a difference between the laboratory and the clinic.

Williams challenges clinicians to ask more meaningful questions which can be followed by systematic observation in the diagnostic and therapeutic situation, as well as in the more formal laboratory. Let us be reminded of Williams' statement, "If the questions for which the researcher seeks answers are not meaningful, then the clinician is at fault for failing to provide the basis for meaningful questions."

These comments coincide appropriately with developments in the field of psychology where the testing of learning principles is giving precision to clinical psychology and where the clinic and the laboratory are losing their distinctiveness. (Wolpe, Salter, and Reyna, 1964; Krasner and Ullman, 1965; Ullman and Krasner, 1965)

In the present volume, Murray's studies, and those investigations by others to which he referred, are examples of making more rigorous and meaningful observations of clinical, therapeutic processes. Efforts to improve the techniques for evaluating speech behavior, such as those discussed by Johnson *et al.* (1961), were intended to be the forerunners of similar therapy studies in the field of speech pathology.

The Iowa contributions, which emphasize "a careful evaluation of our evaluations," are well known. Williams advises the clinician to remember that his evaluation of the problem of stuttering, his "theory about the stuttering," affects what he teaches the client. When the clinician observes behavior, Williams says, he does not merely collect data, he assesses the meaning or significance of it. Unforeseen to him, the clinician sometimes finds on closer examination an incongruity between his techniques and theory.

THERAPEUTIC IMPLICATIONS

There seems to be a steadily developing, and at present rather strong, scientifically based system of learning theory from which can be derived certain general principles and specific techniques that may be utilized in stuttering therapy. At this stage speech pathologists are just beginning research which must prove the utility of these concepts and procedures. I will comment on this type of research in the last section of this summary, but first I wish to draw together in review what the contributors to this symposium have said about the present status of learning theory as related to stuttering therapy.

Extinction and Counterconditioning in Stuttering Therapy

Extinction may be defined as the weakening of a response by not following it with reinforcement (reward or punishment). Counterconditioning is defined as either a change in reinforcement, for example, rewarding a response that has previously been punished, or an extinction which is hastened by the reinforcement of a response displacing the original conditioned response. As was seen, Mowrer suggests that extinction and counterconditioning may be identical processes. He reasons that the situation is not neutral when reward is withheld in extinction.

140

Rather, it involves disappointment, which is a form of punishment. On the other hand, when fear is not confirmed by expected punishment, relief, which is a form of reward, is involved. It may be more precise, concludes Mowrer, to say that unlearning always involves counterconditioning.

Luper, Sheehan, and I describe stuttering therapy as a learning procedure in which the fundamental processes occurring are extinction and/or counterconditioning. I have emphasized the importance of creating an atmosphere in which the client is rewarded for discussing his problem as a means of counterconditioning anxiety which has generalized from the punishment associated with stuttering behavior to the act of talking about it. This is viewed as an essential first step in that part of the therapeutic process aimed toward the modification of mediating attitudinal responses. Luper and I have referred to the extinction of fear, the feeling of relief, which the stutterer experiences when provided with an environment in which stuttering is not punished. Furthermore, we have referred to counterconditioning as the mechanism underlying the benefit the stutterer derives from the reward given for facing a feared word or situation. It is counterconditioning also when the stutterer modifies his response in the presence of certain stimulus cues (sounds, words, situations), as for example in voluntary stuttering and the acquisition of new preparatory sets. In addition, Luper and I have made reference to the way in which modeling (Bandura, 1962) and shaping (Skinner, 1959) are utilized in the instating of a new speech pattern when the stutterer follows the directions, and responds to the reinforcement, of the clinician.

Sheehan's lectures and writings over the years, including his contributions to this symposium, have elucidated the conflict nature of stuttering. He views stuttering therapy as being directed toward the reduction of the approach-avoidance conflict at the five levels of word fear, situation fear, the emotional content of speech, interpersonal relations, and ego protection. In his chapter, he has emphasized that stuttering is not a speech problem per se, but rather a problem of the social presentation of the self, a self-role conflict. Anxiety-reduction, avoidance-reduction type speech therapy is the approach recommended by Sheehan to reduce the fear on the word and situational level of conflict. Again, the basic psychological principle of learning involved would appear to be counterconditioning. Sheehan describes more of a psychotherapeutically oriented therapy for work on the remaining three levels of conflict. He acknowledges the emphasis in therapy, as recommended over the years

141

by Bryngelson, Johnson, and Van Riper, on all five of these levels of conflict. However, Sheehan has made an especially noteworthy contribution to stuttering therapy in his emphasis on the importance of the stutterer working through certain feelings, conflicts, or ideas revolving around his self-esteem, his self-concept, and his relationship with others. His description of the stutterer's adjustment into a new role as a more fluent speaker during the latter stages of therapy is another significant contribution. Sheehan's therapy involves a balance between action-taking, behavior therapy with an emphasis on encouraging new and more adequate responses, and an interview relationship of the traditional psychotherapeutic type in which acceptance, understanding, support, information, and interpretation are provided.

I have described the use of instruction in progressive and differential relaxation, emphasizing the techniques of Jacobson (1938). I have found these procedures beneficial in teaching the stutterer to adjust the tonicity of the body, the speech mechanism in particular, and in bringing about a general reduction of anxiety. Reference is made in my discussion to Wolpe's use of relaxation responses in behavior therapy and his rationale that muscle relaxation has autonomic effects antagonistic to those of anxiety. In Wolpe's therapy, relaxation is one of several responses utilized to reciprocally inhibit anxiety.[7] I view teaching the stutterer relaxation responses as a means of counterconditioning anxiety and tension.

Finally, with reference to extinction and counterconditioning, Luper observes that the process is sometimes inefficient, most probably because the behavior has been learned on a partial reinforcement schedule. This points to our need for more research examining the issue of massed and

7. Wolpe (1958) has used principles of learning in developing this method of psychotherapy known as reciprocal inhibition. The approach is based on the premise that neurotic behavior involves unadaptive, conditioned anxiety (autonomic) responses and, therefore, successful treatment requires the reinforcement of some response, such as relaxation, which reciprocally inhibits the anxiety response. This antagonistic response should be reinforced in the presence of a stimulus that ordinarily generates neurotic anxiety. A desensitization procedure is employed by working on stimulus situations that arouse anxiety, beginning with the least anxiety-evoking and working up the hierarchy to the most anxiety-arousing.

Brutten and Shoemaker (1967) have adapted Wolpe's procedure to stuttering therapy. They utilize reciprocal inhibition to diminish the "conditioned emotional responses that disorganize fluent speech behavior" (Bloodstein and Brutten, 1966, p. 385) and, in addition, they use massed response repetition, aimed toward the accomplishing of reactive and conditioned inhibition, to extinguish avoidance behaviors.

distributed extinction and/or counterconditioning. While experimental evidence is not conclusive, it seems that massed counterconditioning will produce a greater immediate reduction of fear. I have often felt that this was one of the problems in treatment programs for stutterers in the public schools. It may be difficult for a child, with this type of fear-motivated problem, to experience, in twenty or thirty minutes per week, enough change in behavior and the accompanying rewards to counteract the fear and the avoidance behavior which has built up over a period of years.

Generalization

Once a response has been conditioned to a particular stimulus, similar stimuli will tend to evoke the response also. Murray has referred to the way in which this process of generalization operates in the learning of socially unadaptive behavior, and all of the writers on stuttering in this volume have described generalization as it takes place in the development of stuttering. Obviously, therefore, stimulus generalization and its opposite, discrimination, are important considerations in the unlearning and relearning process.

In my chapter I emphasized, as have Miller and Dollard in psychotherapy, the need to correct the generalizations in thinking which occur during the childhood period when stuttering develops. This is accomplished through a cognitive process of verbal labeling. An additional part of the rationale for this procedure is the concept that verbal behavior in the human being is very important as a cue for overt responses. Murray notes the use in psychotherapy of approaches which change the subject's "verbal formulas" for behavior.

Stuttering therapy involves, therefore, the correction of generalization through discrimination; but on the other hand, the phenomena of generalization of extinction and/or counterconditioning help, as Luper has stated, to shorten the process of unlearning and relearning involved in therapy. The clinician can expect the extinction or counterconditioning he has done to spread to other situations that are similar. In this connection, Sheehan has stressed that stuttering is a social relation disorder and that modifications of behavior should be worked on in a group, as well as in individual therapy. I have reported on an open clinic, group therapy approach in which the stutterer's family, friends, and other interested persons (often my students) are encouraged to participate in the discussions and activities of the group sessions. This approach provides an appropriate setting for the practicing of roles representing situations in real life to which the stutterer needs to generalize new behavior. Furthermore, this approach takes into consideration a gradual desensitization approach in which responses are changed, first in the presence of stimuli which evoke minimal anxiety, and then in situations which have a history of producing higher levels of anxiety.

In conclusion, stimulus generalization is an important principle to be considered in stuttering therapy. Most clinicians appear aware of this, but it is my impression that all of the contributors to the symposium felt that greater attention needs to be given to the planning of procedures and situations which take advantage of generalization or bring it about. In terms of concern about therapy in the public schools, this setting offers many excellent opportunities for the generalization of new responses.

THERAPY RESEARCH

During the last fifteen years, speech pathologists have increasingly made references to the need for studies of the process and outcome of speech therapy, including therapy for stutterers. In a special report on "Research Needs in Speech Pathology" published in 1959, Brown, Sheehan, West, and Wischner offered the following statement in commenting on research needs in stuttering:

Although the committee clearly recognizes the difficulties inherent in research designed to evaluate clinical techniques and programs for stutterers, it regards the needs for such research as urgent. (p. 29)

Van Riper has provided some valuable descriptive information on the process, outcome, and follow-up of stuttering therapy in his chapter, "Experiments in Stuttering Therapy," in *Stuttering: A Symposium* (1958). Earlier, Shames (1952, 1953) reported studies investigating the value of certain biographical and personality information in predicting success in therapy. In this research, which involved thirty-seven subjects with four different types of speech problems, the number of variables investigated having a statistically significant relationship with success was less than the number which would be expected by chance. Reporting on group homogeneity and success in speech therapy, Shames suggested that subjects in therapy who are more alike in age, education, socio-economic level, type of problem, and type of social and psychological difficulties will attain on the average greater success than a less

144

homogeneous group. Shames emphasized the exploratory nature and limitations of these studies. He urged that larger samples of one type of speech disorder be studied using a standardized therapeutic climate. Sheehan (1954) evaluated the use of the Rorschach as a prognostic tool in the treatment of stuttering. Predictions based on the Klopfer Prognostic Scale were found useful in predicting psychotherapeutic improvement but could not be used in predicting speech improvement. Williams and Kent (1959) studied the effect of a tranquilizer, meprobamate, as an adjunct to stuttering therapy. They utilized an experimental and a control group, matched on the basis of age, sex, amount of previous therapy, severity ratings, and MMPI profiles. Changes in speech behavior, as evaluated using a seven-point rating scale, revealed no significant differences in change in speech behavior between the two groups.

Another study of a type that I believe to be of considerable importance is the one by Sheehan and Voas (1957), in which they compared the effect on stuttering adaptation of three different techniques of negative practice: (1) initiation of actual stuttering pattern, (2) bounce (syllable repetition), and (3) slide (syllable prolongation). It should be noted that this was not a study of an actual therapy situation, but rather it involved what has been called a laboratory model of a therapy situation. Sheehan concluded that initiating the actual stuttering pattern on purpose significantly retarded adaptation. The bounce and slide techniques appeared to reduce the frequency of stuttering behavior, but no more than standard adaptation readings.

Recently, I have undertaken a three-year study to investigate the results of stuttering therapy with adults when a carefully described approach is used. More specifically, the purpose of the investigation is to study the relationship among changes which occur on certain measured variables, and also the relationship between these changes and certain evaluated characteristics of the individual. Another purpose is to evaluate the follow-up period to see whether changes that occurred in therapy are maintained.

The approach to stuttering therapy which is being evaluated is essentially the avoidance-reduction, anxiety-reduction therapy system, based principally on concepts of learning theory psychology as described over the years by Bryngelson (1950), Johnson (1956), Sheehan (1958b), and Van Riper (1963). The hypotheses (listed below) of the investigation will serve to make clear the fact that the variables one chooses to investigate are a reflection of one's concept of the problem under study.

145

1. There will be a decrement in the severity of stuttering behavior in terms of severity ratings of the tape recordings of reading and speaking samples.

2. Specific speech-associated anxiety will be reduced as measured by palmar sweat prints.

3. There will be a reduction of general anxiety as measured by the Taylor Manifest Anxiety Scale and the Holtzman Inkblot Test.

4. There will be an improvement in certain of the stutterer's personality characteristics, as assessed by the Holtzman Inkblot Test, the Minnesota Multiphasic Personality Inventory, and the Edwards Personal Preference Schedule.

5. Avoidance of speaking situations will be reduced as measured by the Stutterer's Self-Ratings of Reactions to Speech Situations Scale.

6. There will be an improved attitude toward stuttering as measured by the Iowa Scale of Attitude Toward Stuttering.

I am interested in studying a specific approach to stuttering therapy rather than comparing therapies. One might think that the best way to proceed would be to match an experimental group which receives therapy with a control group which does not receive therapy. However, it is readily apparent that it is very difficult to control or equate such variables as type of stuttering, important environmental influences, personality, and socio-economic level. In view of these difficulties, a research design was chosen in which the subjects serve as their own controls. As diagramed below, twenty adult stutterers will be given a battery of tests nine months before therapy begins, again at the beginning of a nine-month therapy period, at the end of the therapy period, and nine months after the close of therapy. This design is based on that used by Rogers and Dymond (1954) in their classic research study of the interrelationships between outcome variables in client-centered therapy.

Prewait Testing	Pretherapy Testing	Post-therapy Testing	Follow-up Testing
Waiting period 9 months	Therapy period 9 months	Follow-up period 9 months	

146

Hopefully, there will be more research studies contrasting periods of no treatment with the periods of treatment, treatment and no-treatment groups, and, where feasible, comparisons of the therapeutic effectiveness of different types of treatment. Without studies like these, it is not possible to make definitive statements about the efficacy of certain types of therapy.

Of course, research on therapy is not simply a matter of testing well-formulated hypotheses. Hypotheses develop from experience in which clinicians explore, and attempt to describe, the variables which can and should be studied. Therefore, I should like to echo Williams, who encouraged clinicians to utilize their experience more fully in carrying out descriptive studies of *what* is happening in therapy. I have encouraged clinicians to think of each subject as a research project and to determine what dependent or criteria variables are to be changed and what independent variables are going to be manipulated. I find that this approach helps clinicians to bridge the supposed gap between clinical work and research. In addition, my experience has indicated that the careful planning and execution of therapy with the increased rigor of a research investigation improves clinical performance.

The outcome studies reviewed at the beginning of this section and the extensive, long-range assessment of the results of stuttering therapy presently in progress at Northwestern University will provide data which are needed; however, in future studies there is also a need to focus on more definitive applications of learning principles in bringing about behavior modifications. The laboratory investigation by Sheehan and Voas (1957) reviewed earlier is of the more specific nature to which I refer. The more recent work of Flanagan, Goldiamond, and Azrin (1958), and Martin and Siegel (1966), studying the effects of response-contingent punishment on stuttering, are additional examples of laboratory studies investigating the effect of a specific influence or variable.[8] Furthermore, research is needed which is aimed toward identifying the individual characteristics of stutterers, such as high or low general anxiety, differential galvanic skin responses, and minimal language or motor deficits that are related to the stutterer's susceptibility to various procedures.

Finally, there is, at this time, a growing tendency for the research-oriented speech pathologist to be more interested in experimental-clinical research in which the learning principles discussed in this volume

8. See Bloodstein and Brutten (1966) for a review of research on punishment and stuttering behavior.

are studied during the assessment and therapy process in the clinic. Brookshire (1967) and Holland (1967) have provided concise reviews of some basic principles of behavior modification which need to be examined with greater precision in the clinic-laboratory situation. Careful investigations are needed of such factors (mentioned by Brookshire and Holland) as the appropriateness and the timing of reinforcement, the gradual and progressive development of a new response utilizing small units, and the extension of stimulus control from the clinic to outside situations. In addition, schedules of reinforcement and the schedules of following conditioned reinforcers with the "back-up reinforcers" (e.g., tokens as conditioned reinforcers and food as back-up reinforcer) need to be studied. On the diagnostic side of clinical research, studies are needed which deal with methods for assessing the stimuli controlling behavior in each individual case, those reinforcements which are most effective, and how best to modify the reinforcing stimuli of the environment.

Bibliography

ALLPORT, G. W. (1935) Attitudes. In C. MURCHISON (Ed.), *Handbook of social psychology*. Worcester, Mass.: Clark University Press.

AMSEL, A. (1958) The role of frustrative nonreward in noncontinuous reward situations. *Psychol. Bull., 55*, 102–19.

ANDREWS, G., and HARRIS, M. (1964) *The syndrome of stuttering*. London: Spastic Society Medical Education and Information Unit, Levenham Press.

ARNOLD, G., and LUCHSINGER, R. (1965) *Voice-speech-language*. Belmont, Calif.: Wadsworth.

BACHRACH, A. J. (1962) *Experimental foundations of clinical psychology*. New York: Basic Books.

BANDURA, A. (1956) Psychotherapist's anxiety level, self-insight, and psychotherapeutic competence. *J. Abnorm. & Soc. Psychol., 52*, 333–37.

———. (1962) Social learning through imitation. In M. R. JONES (Ed.),

Nebraska symposium on motivation. Lincoln, Neb.: University of Nebraska Press.

BARDRICK, R. A., and SHEEHAN, J. G. (1956) Emotional loadings as a source of conflict in stuttering. *Amer. Psychologist, 11,* 391.

BEECH, H. R. (1960) The symptomatic treatment of writer's cramp. In H. J. EYSENCK (Ed.), *Behavior therapy and neuroses.* New York: Pergamon, 349–72.

BERLIN, A. (1954) *An exploratory attempt to isolate types of stuttering.* Ph.D. dissertation, Northwestern University.

BIJOU, S. W., and ORLANDO, R. (1961) Rapid development of multiple schedule performance with retarded children. *J. Exp. Anal. Behav., 4,* 7–16.

BITTERMAN, M. E., FEDDERSEN, W. E., and TYLER, D. W. (1953) Secondary reinforcement and the discrimination hypothesis. *Amer. J. Psychol., 66,* 456–64.

BLOODSTEIN, O. (1958) Stuttering as an anticipatory struggle reaction. In J. EISENSON (Ed.), *Stuttering: a symposium.* New York: Harper.

———, and BRUTTEN, E. J. (1966) Stuttering problems. In R. W. REIBER and R. S. BRUBAKER (Eds.), *Speech pathology.* Amsterdam: North-Holland.

BROOKSHIRE, R. H. (1967) Speech pathology and the experimental analysis of behavior. *J. Speech and Hear. Dis., 32,* 215–27.

BROWN, S. R., SHEEHAN, J. G., WEST, R. W., and WISCHNER, G. J. (1959) Report of subcommittee on the problem of stuttering and problems of rate and fluency. Research needs in speech pathology and audiology. *J. Speech and Hear. Dis., Mono. Supp. 5,* 26–30.

BRUTTEN, E. J., and SHOEMAKER, D. J. (1967) *The modification of stuttering.* Englewood Cliffs, N. J.: Prentice-Hall.

BRYNGELSON, B., *et al.* (1950) *Know yourself: a workbook for those who stutter.* Rev. ed. Minneapolis, Minn.: Burgess.

CHERBONNIER, E. L. (1955) *Hardness of heart.* Garden City, N. Y.: Doubleday.

CURRY, F. K. W., and GREGORY, H. H. (1967) A comparison of stutterers and nonstutterers on three dichotic tasks. Paper read at American Speech and Hearing Association Convention, Chicago, November 1967.

DELACATO, C. H. (1963) *The diagnosis and treatment of speech and reading problems.* Springfield, Ill.: Charles Thomas.

DITTES, J. E. (1957) Extinction during psychotherapy of GSR accompanying "embarrassing" statements. *J. Abnorm. & Soc. Psychol., 54,* 187–91.

DOLLARD, J., and MILLER, N. E. (1950) *Personality and psychotherapy.* New York: McGraw-Hill.

DOLLARD, J., and MOWRER, O. H. (1947) A method of measuring tension in written documents. *J. Abnorm. & Soc. Psychol., 42,* 3–32.

150

EYSENCK, H. J. (Ed.). (1960) *Behavior therapy and the neuroses.* New York: Pergamon.

FARBER, I. E. (1963) The things people say to themselves. *Amer. Psychologist, 18,* 185–87.

FERSTER, C. B. (1961) Positive reinforcement and behavior deficits of autistic children. *Child Developm., 32,* 437–56.

————, and SKINNER, B. F. (1957) *Schedules of reinforcement.* New York: Appleton-Century-Crofts.

FLANAGAN, B., GOLDIAMOND, I., and AZRIN, N. (1958) Operant stuttering: the control of stuttering behavior through response-contingent consequences. *J. Exp. Anal. Behav., 1,* 173–77.

————, ————, ————. (1959) Instatement of stuttering in normally fluent individuals through operant procedures. *Science, 130,* 979–81.

FLAVELL, J. H. (1963) *The developmental psychology of Jean Piaget.* Princeton, N. J.: D. Van Nostrand.

FREDERICK, C. J. (1955) An investigation of learning theory and reinforcement as related to stuttering behavior. Ph.D. dissertation, University of California, Los Angeles.

FREUD, S. (1920) *A general introduction to psychoanalysis.* New York: Liveright.

FRICK, J. V. (1951) An exploratory study of the effect of punishment (electric shock) upon stuttering behavior. Ph.D. dissertation, University of Iowa.

GLAD, D. D. (1959) *Operational values in psychotherapy.* New York: Oxford University Press.

GOLDIAMOND, I. (1965) Stuttering and fluency as manipulatable operant response classes. In L. KRASNER and L. ULLMAN (Eds.), *Research in behavior modification.* New York: Holt, Rinehart & Winston, 106–56.

GOODSTEIN, L. (1958) Functional speech disorders and personality, a survey of the research. *J. Speech and Hear. Res., 1,* 359–76.

GREENSPOON, J. (1955) The reinforcing effect of two spoken sounds on the frequency of two responses. *Amer. J. Psychol., 68,* 409–16.

GREGORY, H. H. (1959) *An investigation of the integrity of the neurophysiological auditory feedback system in stutterers.* Ph.D. dissertation, Northwestern University.

————. (1961) A group social approach to stuttering therapy. *ASHA, 3,* 347 (abstract).

————. (1964a) Stuttering and auditory central nervous system disorder. *J. Speech and Hear. Res., 7,* 335–41.

————. (1964b) Speech clinic helps the adult stutterer. *Rehab. Record, 5,* 9–12.

————. (1965) Applications of learning theory concepts in the management of stuttering. *Acta Societalis Internationalis Logopaediae and Phoniatriae,* *1,* 329–32.

GROSS, M. S., and GREGORY, H. H. (1966) The use of operant conditioning procedures in conjunction with a more traditional stuttering therapy program. Paper read at American Speech and Hearing Association Convention, Washington, November 1966.

————, and NATHANSON, S. N. (1967) A study of the use of a DAF shaping procedure for adult stutterers. Paper read at American Speech and Hearing Association Convention, Chicago, November 1967.

GUTHRIE, E. R. (1952) *The psychology of learning.* Rev. ed. New York: Harper.

GUTTMAN, N., and KALISH, H. I. (1956) Discriminability and stimulus generalization. *J. Exp. Psychol., 51,* 79–88.

HELLER, K. (1963) Experimental analogues of psychotherapy: the clinical relevance of laboratory findings of social influence. *J. Ner. and Ment. Dis., 137,* 420–26.

HILL, W. R. (1963) *Learning: a survey of psychological interpretations.* San Francisco: Chandler.

HOLLAND, A. (1967) Some applications of behavioral principles to clinical speech problems. *J. Speech and Hear. Dis., 32,* 11–18.

HOLT, E. B. (1931) *Animal drive and the learning process.* Vol. I. New York: Henry Holt.

HONIG, W. K. (1961) Generalization of extinction on the spectral continuum. *Psychol. Record, 11,* 267–78.

HULL, C. L. (1943) *Principles of behavior.* New York: Appleton-Century-Crofts.

HUMPHREYS, L. G. (1939a) Acquisition and extinction of verbal expectations in a situation analogous to conditioning. *J. Exp. Psychol., 25,* 294–301.

————. (1939b) The effect of random alternation of reinforcement on the acquisition and extinction of conditioned eyelid reactions. *J. Exp. Psychol., 25,* 141–58.

JACOBSON, E. (1938) *Progressive relaxation.* Chicago: University of Chicago Press.

JOHNSON, W. (1946) *People in quandaries.* New York: Harper.

————. (1955) *Stuttering in children and adults.* Minneapolis, Minn.: University of Minnesota Press.

————, et al. (1956) *Speech handicapped school children.* New York: Harper.

————, et al. (1961) Studies of speech disfluency and rate of stutterers and nonstutterers. *J. Speech and Hear. Dis., Mono. Supp. 7.*

JOURARD, S. (1964) *The transparent self.* Princeton, N.J.: D. Van Nostrand.

152

KIMBLE, G. (1961) *Hilgard and Marquis' conditioning and learning.* New York: Appleton-Century-Crofts.

KRASNER, L. (1958) Studies of the conditioning of verbal behavior. *Psychol. Bull., 55,* 148–70.

———. (1961) The therapist as a social reinforcement machine. In H. H. STRUPP (Ed.), *Second research conference on psychotherapy.* Chapel Hill, N. C.: American Psychological Association, 61–94.

———, and ULLMAN, L. P. (1965) *Research in behavior modification.* New York: Holt, Rinehart & Winston.

LEWIN, K. (1936) *Principles of topological psychology.* New York: McGraw-Hill.

LUPER, H. L. (1956) Consistency of stuttering in relation to the goal gradient hypothesis. *J. Speech and Hear. Dis., 21,* 336–42.

———, and MULDER, R. L. (1964) *Stuttering: therapy for children.* Englewood Cliffs, N. J.: Prentice-Hall.

MARTIN, R. R., and SIEGEL, G. M. (1966) The effects of response contingent shock on stuttering. *J. Speech and Hear. Res., 9,* 340–52.

MEAD, G. H. (1934) *Mind, self, and society.* Chicago: University of Chicago Press.

MILLER, N. E. (1944) Experimental studies of conflict. In J. McV. HUNT (Ed.), *Personality and the behavior disorders.* Vol. I. New York: Ronald Press, 431–65.

———. (1963) Some reflections on the law of effect produce a new alternative to drive reduction. In M. R. JONES (Ed.), *Nebraska symposium on motivation.* Lincoln, Neb.: University of Nebraska Press, 65–112.

———. (1964) Some implications of modern behavior therapy for personality change and psychotherapy. In P. WORCHEL and D. BYRNE (Eds.), *Personality change.* New York: John Wiley, 149–75.

MOWRER, O. H. (1939) A stimulus-response analysis of anxiety and its role as a reinforcing agent. *Psychol. Rev., 46,* 553–65.

———. (1945) Habit strength as a function of the pattern of reinforcement. *J. Exp. Psychol., 35,* 293–311.

———. (1948) Learning theory and the neurotic paradox. *Amer. J. Orthopsychiat., 18,* 571–610.

———. (1956) Two-factor learning theory reconsidered, with special reference to secondary reinforcement and the concept of habit. *Psychol. Rev., 63,* 114–28.

———. (1960a) *Learning theory and behavior.* New York: John Wiley.

———. (1960b) *Learning theory and the symbolic processes.* New York: John Wiley.

———. (1961) *The crisis in psychiatry and religion.* Princeton, N. J.: D. Van Nostrand.

Mowrer, O. H. (1964) *The new group therapy*. Princeton, N.J.: D. Van Nostrand.

————. (1965a) Behavior therapies with special reference to modeling and imitation. Paper presented at Gutheil Memorial Conference, Association for the Advancement of Psychotherapy, New York, October 31, 1965.

————. (1965b) Learning theory and behavior therapy. In B. Wolman (Ed.), *Handbook of clinical psychology*. New York: McGraw-Hill.

————. (1965c) *Morality and mental health*. Chicago: Rand McNally.

————. (1967) Stuttering as simultaneous admission and denial. *J. Communication Dis., 1*, 46–50.

————, and Jones, H. M. (1945) Habit strength as a function of the pattern of reinforcement. *J. Exp. Psychol., 35*, 293–311.

————, and Ullman, A. D. (1945) Time as a determinant of integrative learning. *Psychol. Rev., 52*, 61–90.

Murray, E. J. (1954) A case study in a behavioral analysis of psychotherapy. *J. Abnorm. & Soc. Psychol., 49*, 305–10.

————. (1956) A content-analysis method for studying psychotherapy. *Psychol. Mono., 70* (Whole No. 420).

————. (1962) Direct analysis from the viewpoint of learning theory. *J. Consult. Psychol., 26*, 226–31.

————. (1964) Sociotropic-learning approach to psychotherapy. In P. Worchel and D. Byrne (Eds.), *Personality change*. New York: John Wiley, 249–88.

————, Auld, R., and White, A. M. (1954) A psychotherapy case showing progress but no decrease in the discomfort-relief quotient. *J. Consult. Psychol., 18*, 349–53.

Osgood, C. E. (1953) *Method and theory in experimental psychology*. New York: Oxford University Press.

Pavlov, I. P. (1927) *Conditioned reflexes*. C. V. Anrep (trans.). London: Oxford University Press.

Perkins, W. H. (1967) Modification of stuttering by rate control. (Mimeographed report.) Los Angeles: University of Southern California, Vocational Rehabilitation Administration Planning Grant RD-2180-S, August 1967.

Rogers, C. R. (1942) *Counseling and psychotherapy*. Boston: Houghton Mifflin.

————. (1951) *Client-centered therapy*. Boston: Houghton Mifflin.

————, and Dymond, R. F. (1954) *Psychotherapy and personality change*. Chicago: University of Chicago Press.

Rosenthal, D. (1955) Changes in some moral values following psychotherapy. *J. Consult. Psychol., 19*, 431–36.

Rutherford, D. R. (1963) Personal communication.

Ryan, B. P., and Shames, G. H. (1966) The construction and evaluation of a program for modifying stuttering behavior employing operant conditioning principles. Paper read at American Speech and Hearing Association Convention, Washington, November 1966.

ST. ONGE, R. R. (1963) The stuttering syndrome. *J. Speech and Hear. Res.,* 6, 195–97.

SAPOLSKY, A. (1960) Effect of interpersonal relationships upon verbal conditioning. *J. Abnorm. & Soc. Psychol.,* 60, 241–46.

SARBIN, T. R. (1943) The concept of role taking. *Sociometry,* 6, 273–385.

————. (1954) Role theory. In G. LINDZEY (Ed.), *Handbook of social psychology.* Cambridge, Mass.: Addison-Wesley, 223–58.

SHAMES, G. H. (1952) An investigation of prognosis and evaluation in speech therapy. *J. Speech and Hear. Dis.,* 17, 386–92.

————. (1953) An exploration of group homogeneity in group speech therapy. *J. Speech and Hear. Dis.,* 18, 267–72.

————, and SHERRICK, C. E. (1963) A discussion of non-fluency and stuttering as operant behavior. *J. Speech and Hear. Dis.,* 28, 3–18.

SHEARER, W. M., and WILLIAMS, J. D. (1965) Self-recovery from stuttering. *J. Speech and Hear. Dis.,* 30, 288–90.

SHEEHAN, J. G. (1951) The modification of stuttering through non-reinforcement. *J. Abnorm. & Soc. Psychol.,* 46, 51–63.

————. (1953a) The theory and treatment of stuttering as an approach-avoidance conflict. *J. Psychol.,* 36, 27–49.

————. (1953b) Rorschach changes during psychotherapy in relationship to the personality of the therapist. *Amer. Psychologist,* 8, 434–35.

————. (1954) An integration of psychotherapy and speech therapy through a conflict theory of stuttering. *J. Speech and Hear. Dis.,* 19, 474–82.

————. (1958a) Projective studies of stuttering. *J. Speech and Hear. Dis.,* 23, 18–25.

————. (1958b) Conflict theory of stuttering. In J. EISENSON (Ed.), *Stuttering: a symposium.* New York: Harper, 123–66.

————. (1960) *Research frontiers in stuttering.* (Mimeographed.) UCLA Psychology Speech Clinic.

———— (Ed.). (1968) *Stuttering: research and therapy.* New York: Harper & Row.

————, CORTESE, P., and HADLEY, R. (1962) Guilt, shame, and tension in graphic projections of stuttering. *J. Speech and Hear. Dis.,* 27, 129–39.

————, HADLEY, R. and GOULD, E. (1967) Impact of authority on stuttering. *J. Abnorm. Psychol.,* 72, 290–93.

————, and MARTYN, M. M. (1966) Spontaneous recovery from stuttering. *J. Speech and Hear. Res.,* 9, 121–35.

————, and VOAS, R. B. (1957) Stuttering as conflict: I. Comparison of therapy techniques involving approach-avoidance. *J. Speech and Hear. Dis.,* 22, 714–23.

155

SKINNER, B. F. (1938) *The behavior of organisms.* New York: Appleton-Century-Crofts.

———. (1948) "Superstition" in the pigeon. *J. Exp. Psychol., 38,* 162–72.

———. (1953) *Science and human behavior.* New York: Macmillan.

———. (1957a) The experimental analysis of behavior. *Amer. Scien., 45,* 343–71.

———. (1957b) *Verbal behavior.* New York: Appleton-Century-Crofts.

———. (1959) *Cumulative record.* New York: Appleton-Century-Crofts.

Speech Foundation of America. (1960) *Stuttering and its treatment.* Memphis, Tenn.: M. Fraser.

———. (1962) *Stuttering: its prevention.* Memphis, Tenn.: M. Fraser.

———. (1964) *Treatment of the young stutterer in the school.* Memphis, Tenn.: M. Fraser.

———. (1966) *Stuttering: training the therapist.* Memphis, Tenn.: M. Fraser.

STAATS, A. W., and STAATS, C. V. (1964) *Complex human behavior.* New York: Holt, Rinehart & Winston.

THORNDIKE, E. L. (1931) *Human learning.* New York: Appleton-Century-Crofts.

———. (1932) *The fundamentals of learning.* New York: Teachers College, Columbia University.

———. (1935) *The psychology of wants, interests and attitudes.* New York: Appleton-Century-Crofts.

ULLMAN, L. P., and KRASNER, L. (Eds.). (1965) *Case studies in behavior modification.* New York: Holt, Rinehart & Winston.

VAN RIPER, C. (1947, 1954, 1963) *Speech correction: principles and methods.* 2d ed., 3d ed., 4th ed. Englewood Cliffs, N. J.: Prentice-Hall.

———. (1958) Experiments in stuttering therapy. In J. EISENSON (Ed.), *Stuttering: a symposium.* New York: Harper.

———. (1968) A brief history of the treatment of stuttering. In J. G. SHEEHAN (Ed.), *Stuttering: research and therapy.* New York: Harper & Row.

WALVOORD, B. B., and HALL, H. P. (1966) *Help wanted; a guidebook for parents and therapists dealing with young nonfluent children.* Evanston, Ill.: Northwestern University Speech Clinic.

WATSON, J. B. (1914) *Behavior: an introduction to comparative psychology.* New York: Henry Holt.

———. (1919) *Psychology from the standpoint of a behaviorist.* Philadelphia: J. B. Lippincott.

WILLIAMS, D. E. (1957) A point of view about stuttering. *J. Speech and Hear. Dis., 22,* 390–97.

———, and KENT, L. R. (1959) Use of meprobamate as an adjunct to stuttering therapy. *J. Speech and Hear. Dis., 24,* 64–69.

WINGATE, M. E. (1964) Recovery from stuttering. *J. Speech and Hear. Dis.*, *29*, 312–21.

————. (1966a) Stuttering adaptation and learning: I. The relevance of adaptation studies to stuttering as learned behavior. *J. Speech and Hear. Dis.*, *31*, 148–56.

————. (1966b) Stuttering adaptation and learning: II. The adequacy of learning principles in the interpretation of stuttering. *J. Speech and Hear. Dis.*, *31*, 211–18.

WISCHNER, G. J. (1950) Stuttering behavior and learning: a preliminary theoretical formulation. *J. Speech and Hear. Dis.*, *15*, 324–35.

————. (1952a) Anxiety reduction as reinforcement in maladaptive behavior: evidence in stutterers' representations of the moment of difficulty. *J. Abnorm. Soc. & Psychol.*, *47*, 566–71.

————. (1952b) An experimental approach to expectancy and anxiety in stuttering behavior. *J. Speech and Hear. Dis.*, *17*, 139–54.

————. (1965) Stuttering behavior and the development of stuttering: a review and evaluation of theoretical formulations based on principles of learning. Paper delivered at Symposium on principles of learning and the management of stuttering. Evanston, Ill.: Northwestern University.

WOLPE, J. (1958) *Psychotherapy by reciprocal inhibition.* Stanford, Calif.: Stanford University Press.

————, SALTER, A., and REYNA, L. J. (1964) *The conditioning therapies.* New York: Holt, Rinehart & Winston.

WOODWORTH, R. S. (1958) *Dynamics of behavior.* New York: Henry Holt.

ZENER, C. (1937) The significance of behavior accompanying conditioned salivary secretion for theories of the conditioned response. *Amer. J. Psychol.*, *50*, 385–403.

Index

Avoidance behavior: counterconditioning of, 117–20; extinction of, 117–
20; labeled, 117, 118
Avoidance learning, 6, 7; and facilitation of behavior, 8; and independent
stimuli, 8; and inhibition of behavior,
8; and response-correlated stimuli, 8

Behavior: deficits of, 135; inappropriate,
135
Behavior model, 137–38
Behavior therapist, speech clinician as,
137
Behaviorism, 4
Beliefs of the client, 65–66
Bloodstein, O.: and anticipatory struggle
hypothesis, 108; and multiple origin
concept, 108
Brookshire, R. H., on behavior modifi-
cation, 148
Brutten, E. J., on stuttering therapy,
142n.

Cancellation, 120
Classical conditioning: diagram of, 13;
as stimulus substitution, 4; and two-
factor theory, 13, 130
Client: beliefs of, 65–66; identification
of, with therapist, 39
Clinic and laboratory, 139, 140
Clinician: attitude of, 139; basic beliefs
of, 56–61; contrasted with theoretician, 54–56; cooperation of, with
researcher, 54; evaluations of, 58,
59; and research, 53, 54; responsibilities of, 54–56; role of, 139
Clinician's beliefs: and meaning
attached to client's behavior, 59; and
techniques used, 57–61
Conditioned inhibition, 118n.
Conditioning: aversive, 50; classical, 4,
13, 130; higher-order, 9; instrumental,
4, 6; operant, 131–33; respondent,
131; respondent-operant overlap in,
139
Conflict: approach-avoidance, 26, 74–
78; Miller's studies of, 27; and negative therapeutic effect, 33; recognition
of, in therapy, 48–49; self-role, 72,
73; and sex anxiety, 26; and stuttering, 72, 73; treatment of, in therapy,
48–49
Conflict hypothesis, 76–77

Content analysis, 41; categories of, 28–
29; statements about therapist in, 43;
and study of psychotherapy, 28
Counterconditioning, 135, 136; of anxiety, 122; defined, 16, 98; inefficiency
of, 142–43; of inhibited verbal responses, 113; and reciprocal inhibition, 122; in therapy, 98–101
Cue, 22, 130

Defense reactions, 33
Delayed auditory feedback and altered
speech pattern, 123–24
Desensitization, 120, 144
Dewey, J., 4
Discomfort Relief Quotient, 35–36
Discrimination, 143; in therapy, 115
Disfluent speech: causes of, 92; and
environmental variables, 107–8; and
excess tension, 92; fear related to,
109; not always punishing, 92; punishment of, 92; and subject variables,
107–8
Dollard, J.: analysis of learning, 72; on
generalization, 143; theory reviewed,
135–36; on verbal labeling, 143
Drive, 22, 130; decremental, 12; incre-
mental, 12; learned, 24; and learned
anxiety, 24, 109, 130; primary, 8;
secondary 8, 9, 10

External stimuli, 130
Extinction, 132, 135; of anxiety and
PGSR, 37–38; defined, 15–16, 98; of
fear drive, 136; inefficiency of, 142–
43; of inhibited verbal responses, 113;
and intermittent reinforcement, 17–
19; occurring in therapy, 47; and
punishment, 140–41; and recovery
from stuttering, 78; and relief, 140–
41; response, 23; in therapy, 98–101
Evaluations of the clinician, 58, 59

Facilitation of response, 12
Fear: attached to previously neutral
stimuli, 6, 6n.; and avoidance, 6, 7,
8; conditioning, 6, 7; derived from
pain, 20; and drive increase, 11; as
emotion guiding behavior, 15; extinction of, 34–37, 98–99, 113, 119, 136,
141–43; generalization of, 95; of
hesitant speech, 111; learned, 26; as
learned drive, 130; as motivating repression, 24; as psychophysiological

Murray, E. J.: on client-clinician relationship, 38–48; on clinical research, 140; on content analysis studies, 28–33; on generalization, 143

Negative practice, 127; and reactive inhibition, 118n.; use of, in therapy, 117–18
Negative therapeutic effect, 33
Neurotic, contrasted with sociopath, 69
Non-reinforcement, study of, 77–79

Open clinic approach: and counterconditioning, 125; and extinction, 125; and generalization, 125
Operant conditioning, 131–33
Osgood, C. E., on sequential learning, 88

Pavlov, I. P.: and behavioristic view, 4; on classical conditioning, 4 (diagram), 13, 130; on conditioned reflexes, 4; on counterconditioning, 16; on extinction, 15–16; on higher-order conditioning, 9; and motivation, 8; on stimulus-substitution learning, 4, 8
Phobia, as anxiety reaction, 24
Piaget, J., on cognitive development, 126
Place learning: and approach avoidance, 10; related to fear, 10; related to hope, 10
Psychomotor speech pattern: alteration of, 123–24; and use of DAF, 123–24
Psychopathology, as anxiety-reducing responses, 24
Psychotherapy: as anxiety extinction, 39; and verbal behavior, 135–36
Pull-out, 104, 120
Punishment: associated with disfluencies, 92; and avoidance learning, 14; and conditioning of fear, 14; in development of stuttering, 6n.; and inhibition, 14; reduction of, 96, 97; and response-correlated stimuli, 7; as stamping-out, 5; of stuttering, 80, 139; verbal statement and, 41

Reactive inhibition, 118n.
Reinforcement, 130; by anxiety reduction, 131; appropriateness of, 148; in development of stuttering, 6n.; differences in pattern of, 79–80; diminished frustration and, 19; effective-

ness of, 19, 113; environmental, 104; by fear reduction, 8, 102, 103; feedback as, 104; feelings as, 104; gradient of, 23, 102–4; and Greenspoon effect, 40; listener reaction as, 104; negative, 99, 132; partial, 99; positive, 132; by posture change, 40; related to fear reduction, 77; schedules of, 99, 133; secondary, 9, 10, 130; self, 99; social, 99; of stuttering, 75–76, 99, 102, 103, 104; timing of, 148; variable schedule of 99, 102; verbal, 40, 41, 43
Reinforcer: negative, 132; positive, 132
Relaxation: and anxiety reduction, 122–23; autonomic effects of, 122, 142; and counterconditioning anxiety, 142; progressive and differential, 122–23; rationale for, 122–23
Repression: Freudian description of, 68; motivated by fear, 24; related to inhibition, 24
Response, 22, 130; extinction of, 23; facilitation of, 12; generalization of, 23; inhibition of, 12; mediating attitudes as, 110, 111. See also Speech response
Response-correlated stimuli: and fear, 11; and hope, 11; and inhibition, 7; and punishment, 7; and secondary reinforcement, 10
Reward, 22; and external stimuli, 11; and response-produced stimuli, 11; of stuttering, 80; verbal, related to social motive, 43; verbal statement of, 41, 42, 43
Role, as expressed in stuttering, 81
Role-demand study, 73–74
Role theory, 73–74
Role variable: conflict of, 73; related to stuttering, 73; and relationship-level conflict, 74; and self variable, 73; and stuttering therapy, 74
Rosen, J., 30n., 43, 44

Scientific method, 60–61
Secondary drives and two-factor theory, 8, 9, 19
Secondary reinforcement and response-correlated stimuli, 10
Self-concept: of being handicapped, 97; as expressed in stuttering, 81; and stuttering therapy, 74. See also Self variable